THROUGH THE EYES
OF A MASTER

THROUGH THE EYES OF A MASTER

Michelle V. Barnes

ISBN: 1539459446
ISBN 13: 9781539459446
Library of Congress Control Number: 2016916978
CreateSpace Independent Publishing Platform
North Charleston, South Carolina

DEDICATION

I have dedicated my life to Jesus, and so I dedicate my first book to him as well. A dream that was pressed on my heart as a young teenager came to fruition through his gentle nudges, telling me I was capable and good enough to write this book. I pressed into him for knowledge, truth, titles, designs, connections in the book world, and, most important, confidence. As my ego tried aggressively to talk me out of it, he stood over me and told me I could do it. As usual, he was right, and I thank him for that.

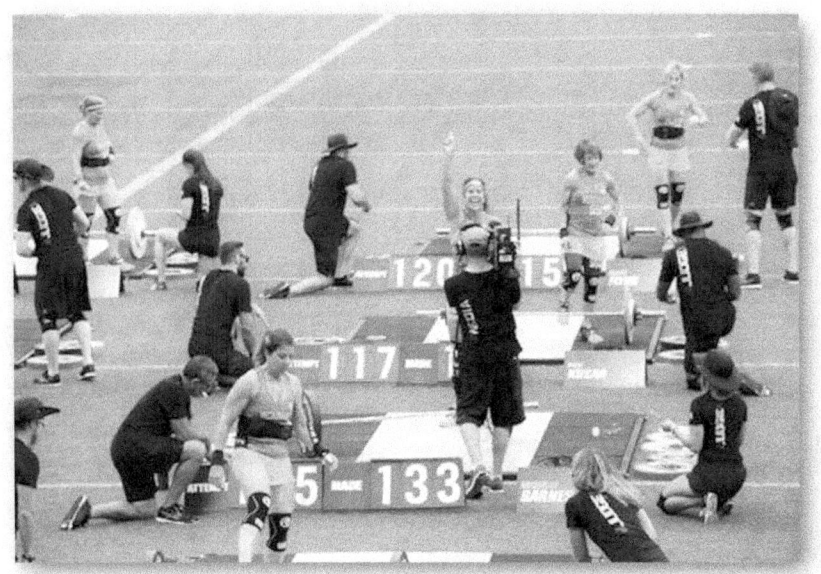

Giving God all the glory after winning an event at the 2015 CrossFit Games.

TABLE OF CONTENTS

PREFACE

THE WORLD WE work, play, and exercise in today is no longer a healthy environment. The battle is on, now more than ever, to preserve our health through abundant God-given nutrition, functional movement, detoxification, positive thoughts, and spirituality. Have you ever dived into this arena, only to become overwhelmed and lacking in hope? Take heed—I am here to tell you that it's your ego playing with you. There is hope, and with a little work—plus knowledge—making changes in your health will soon become your successful destiny. You will encounter journeys and realizations, and you will see things you never knew were possible for others or you. Allow me to take you through my two CrossFit Games. CrossFit is a functional fitness program that anyone can do at any fitness level, all the way to a world-class level. This was an opportunity I stumbled on while trying to find my way to bring my own fitness and nutrition to higher levels.

This book asserts that becoming fit and healthy can be simply interpreted and structured into anyone's lifestyle. Lacking positive motivation will no longer be a question or reality in your mind. I wrote this book because I wanted to share with you that you can and will be better prepared to step up your health in a multifaceted style. Most important, know that these methods are not rocket-scientist designs but necessary and easy enough for beating sickness and disease. Anyone can do this, regardless of age or disabilities.

Learn CrossFit competitive-training secrets as I hold back nothing. You might want to compete in a sport or even CrossFit. CrossFit's benefits cross over into all aspects of your life. If you are yearning for a change in your life, it's more than likely health-related restlessness. So let us begin the journey together, and let's not forget to enjoy the journey.

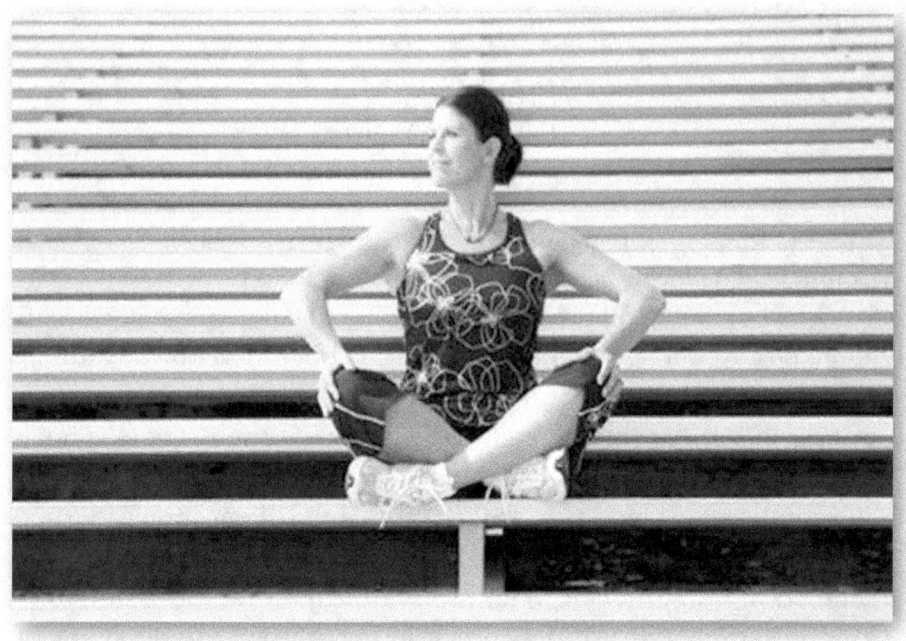

For nothing will be impossible with God ~ Luke 1:37.

CHAPTER 1

THE IMPACT OF YOUR CHILDHOOD ENVIRONMENT

BEING BORN AND raised in Alaska has had its advantages and disadvantages. Where you are born and how you are raised can really have an effect on your life—in both mind and body. My parents moved to Alaska when they were very young and were looking for golden opportunities in both the outdoors and the professional world.

They bore five children in Alaska, and I am the second oldest. For the most part, we grew up with a very active lifestyle. Participating in sports and outdoor recreation such as skiing, running, cycling, canoeing, fishing, softball, basketball, camping, hiking, gardening, and hunting was the norm. I think if you have not been burned out on what you grew up with at a young age—and if it was good stuff—it can be your mold for a healthy lifestyle. You will automatically gravitate toward it, or perhaps you never left it. It is easier to go back into it because it's in you already.

Then there were times when we could not even get out of the house to go to school, let alone participate in an outdoor activity. The ice fog could be thick for several weeks, combined with temperatures well into the sixty-below range, so leaving the house was not an option. My mom would have to take a taxi to the grocery store because the car would not start. If it was plugged in and it started, we could not turn it off in the parking lot while she was shopping because it would not start up again. They didn't have plugs there to keep the engine block from freezing up. Your tires felt like concrete blocks, going *thump* and *thump*! If your car broke down, you could imagine all the terrible things that would apply. It was safer to take the taxi.

The summers are short in Alaska because of poor weather and light availability, causing short sport seasons. As a youngster, I was able to be active, but I never really was given the chance to see that I had lots of athletic ability. This was for a couple of different reasons, but I don't look back at it as anything negative. I know I am where I am today because this is where God has put me. I grew up in a good time in Alaska. It was virgin territory. It's a lot different there now, and I feel blessed to have grown up there during that time.

It is difficult and costly to purchase fresh and healthy food from the grocery stores in Alaska. Although the variety has improved over the years, the prices are still crazy high. By the time the fresh fruit and vegetables reach the grocery shelves, most of the food value is gone because it takes so long after harvest to hit the shelves. My family avoided a lot of these problems by hunting and fishing, and Dad always planted a massive garden during the short summer months. The garden would grow rapidly because of all the extra daylight during this time of year. He would always put up game meat and fish in the freezer, which would last us all year.

When I was a small child, my parents taught me how to become self-sufficient in growing and hunting my own food. It was healthier, less costly, and a valuable tool to learn. Growing your own garden guarantees you that there are no chemicals added in the form of pesticides and fertilizers—deadly chemicals to steer clear of. We also had a chicken coop. There is no comparison to having your own fresh eggs, knowing that what you fed those chickens and allowing them exercise produced healthy eggs. We would can and freeze lots of vegetables and store homegrown potatoes under the house all winter long. We also raised bees, which provided us with our own supply of honey. I was fortunate to have parents who provided for us in a way that taught us how to be healthy from a very young age. I'm pretty sure I complained about being required to do the legwork and requested a bag of Doritos in my lunch every now and then.

One thing I recall doing almost every year was wrapping meat. That was a huge chore. But that's how we rolled, wrapping and marking the meat with the cut type.

My grandmother, Bertha, was considered a health food nut because she grew her own food by raising acres of food and chickens in Washington. My brother still lives on her property today, still raising food. It's one of the few homes in that neighborhood that still has acreage. She also was savvy about taking supplements and juicing. She made sure we always had top-quality vitamins as children. To this day, I am still taking high-quality vitamins and minerals along with many more supplements my body requires. My parents continued her ways. During the summers, I got to fly out from Alaska to Washington to stay on her farm with her.

I learned a lot from my grandparents. Bertha retired from the state of Washington after a career of teaching mentally disabled women to sew. She was loaded with patience and could do about anything she set her mind to. Men could not hang with her. She would work them too hard if she wasn't working circles around them. She had many husbands and finally gave up on men.

I would go with her to work. When we came home from work, she would head out to the chicken coop with her white uniform still on and tear the head off a chicken before throwing the body in a pot of boiling water. My job was to pluck it. That was our dinner, along with fresh vegetables from the garden. If we had bread, it was because she made it.

My grandmother lived to be ninety-nine, and her father, my great-grandfather, lived into his late nineties. They both exercised to Jack LaLanne. She used an inversion table and would stand on her head, back against the front door, for long periods. I also remember her jumping on a rebounder, which looked and acted like a mini trampoline. She even bought my parents a rebounder, which I jumped on in my late teens. I believe so much of that longevity is due to good, healthy living. She never did purchase a microwave oven when they came out. She was dead set against them and fast-food restaurants, too. How is it that she knew how dangerously unhealthy microwaves and fast foods were with only a high school education? I think it's because there is nothing complicated about it. Real food is where the food value is not processed, made-up food.

Our society today is becoming more aware of how important it is to make healthy choices rather than making choices out of a concern for cost or convenience. We're going back to the basics and getting away from chemicals in various forms. Growing up in an environment in which my family made healthy choices was just a way of life for me. It does take a lot of discipline for many people, partly because they did not grow up with it or because it's easier to go for the convenient items. It's important to share with as many people as I can how important it is to make healthy choices and also how to go about it, so we can be happy with the quality of our lives. Many people give up on taking care of themselves way too easily. For some, it's the lack of knowledge. You don't have to be a rocket scientist to eat clean and find a way to exercise. I know it can be extremely challenging for those who were not brought up with a healthy lifestyle, but once you get past the mental part of it and understand the education and results behind it, it's easy to stay on track and reap the rewards. It makes a huge difference in how you feel, and you look and stay healthy. Beating disease before it arrives is the winner here. There is no such thing about reaching retirement and riding off into the sunset doing nothing. You have to work on staying vibrant every day.

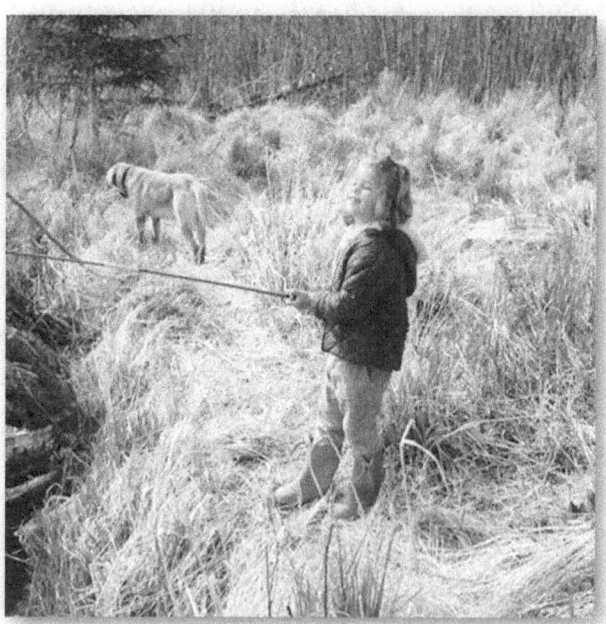

Here I am five years old fishing on the bank of
an Alaskan River with our dog North.

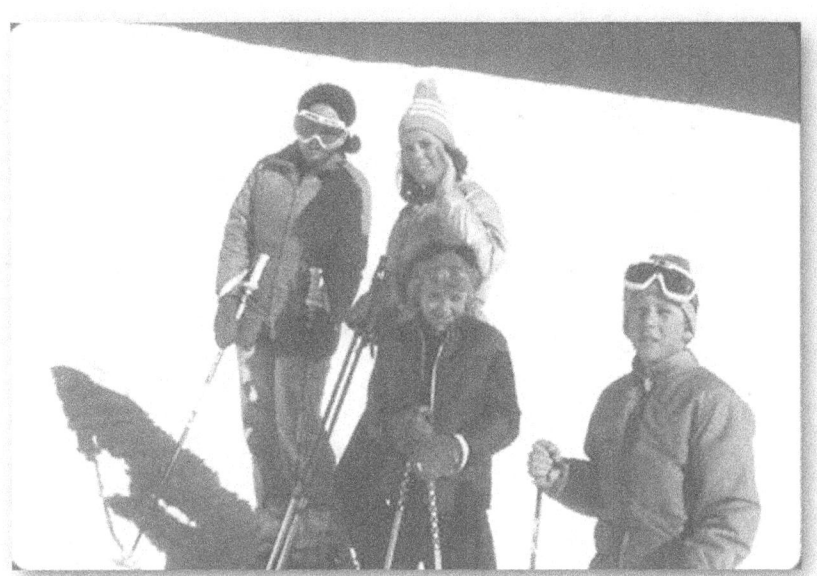

Every weekend we skied together as a family and entered all the races.

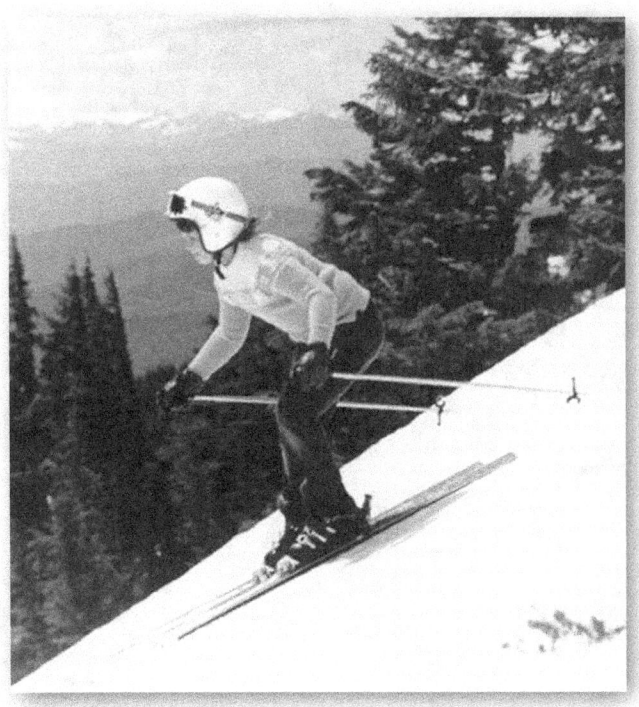

Attending a ski camp in Oregon.

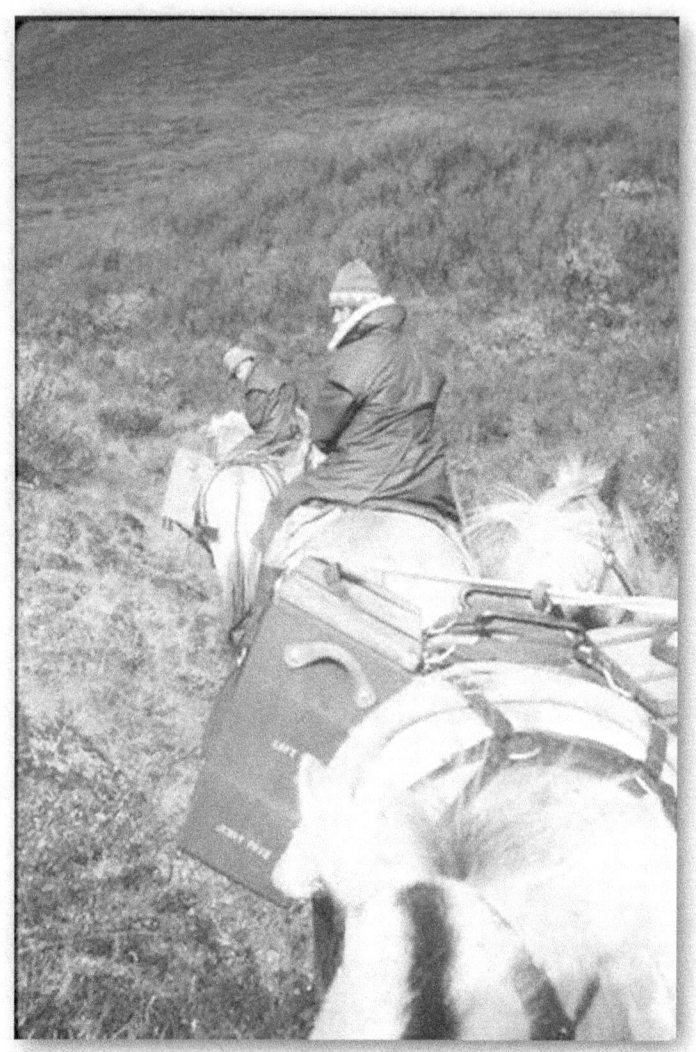

My Dad and I on a hunting trip in Alaska.

CHAPTER 2

MENTAL TOUGHNESS

IF YOU ARE blessed enough to have been raised in an active, positive, and healthy lifestyle, you are well on your way to having developed pieces of what it takes to maintain your health and go into aging healthy. Don't worry if your environment was not so appeasing. Change is all how we receive it. Believe first, and then receive.

Knowing your body both mentally and physically will be to your advantage in many areas. Pay attention to it, as it does tell you information 24/7. Trying to get back into improving your health or striving for optimal health requires mental toughness. It can be like giving your brain a tough workout. The more you do it, the tougher and stronger your discipline becomes. Consistency is a huge key factor. Make it happen.

Try to get into the habit of responding to your body when it is telling you something, rather than ignoring it. It may save your life someday. Plus, many other benefits arise when you listen and pay attention to what your body is telling you. For example, imagine that you feel hungry. Are you actually hungry, or is it a certain stress that is causing you to feel as if you're hungry? If it truly is hunger pangs, think about the last time you ate, and maybe eat a healthy snack if it's time. That's listening to your body and brain and then following through with mental toughness (discipline in making a good choice). For some, this is not an issue; for others, breaking old habits and retraining the brain can be challenging at first. I promise it becomes easier, and soon you will realize the upside of making healthy choices and will not want to go backward. You will become aware that it is not worth it in more ways than one.

Mentality plays a huge part that can affect so many areas of our lives. Approaching everything with a positive attitude is the ultimate goal, but when things go wrong, that can be a challenge for many. Keep searching for something positive, even under negative circumstances. When people thwart negative energy your way, rebound it by responding with positive energy. You can change them sometimes—all while keeping your positive vibe on. I do believe that our world has a ton of negative energy. Just turn the TV on and listen. I refuse to allow the negative energy to affect me as much as possible. I pull out my mental toughness, find the positive energy, and share it. When a positive person walks into the room, you will know it. The same could be said for negative people. Look at their postures, listen to their voices, and engage in their body language. It's easy to see who the Debbie Downer is pretty quickly. I have also found many negative people do not want your input if you will not join them in their negative fest. Usually, they'll go and find someone else who will condone their negative behavior once they conclude you will not. That's a win-win, especially for you! You stay bright and full of love and project vibrant energy, and they take their Negative Nancy attitude with them and move on. You have offered them love through positivity, answers, and solutions, and now it is up to them.

If you have baggage from the past, you've got to face it and get rid of it. It will cost you greatly if you don't. Some folks don't even know they have baggage because they have blocked it out to protect themselves from pain, or they're in denial and don't want to deal with it head-on. I would say if you keep failing at something for some reason or another—like, say, trying to start a better eating habit—then perhaps it's time to dig deeper and find out what may be causing the problem from a mental standpoint. You may be using food for comfort rather than dealing with the situation. A visit to a psychologist may be worth its weight in gold. Food is our primary source of fuel, and it shouldn't be confused with comfort.

I have gained my cleansing through Christ. I have done some counseling and read a lot of self-help books, but I found that Christ never leaves my side, and I can always depend on him. The more time I spend with him, the closer I become with him in our relationship, exposing a treasure chest of gifts he has for me. This has allowed me to work through some childhood issues, as well as day-by-day issues now. You can always find the positive mental toughness in Christ, and yes, sometimes you will have to dig deeper than other times. A good pastor can help you obtain that deep, personal relationship with Christ. You can even ask a friend you know who has a mature Christian persona.

I received Christ as my Lord and Savior as a very young child. It wasn't until I was in my late thirties that I began to understand the love he had for me. At that point, I started spending quality time with him. When my relationship with him began to mature, it became obvious to me that he was without a doubt my help in mental toughness. There is nothing I go through without him now. It has not always been that way. My growth with him has come in the form of trials and tribulations. As the years have passed by, he has become my rock, my fortress. I cannot imagine my life without him. I wish for everyone to receive this free gift.

Surrounding yourself with people who are positive and upbeat will make a positive difference in your quality of life. Negative people can be extremely draining and do more damage than good. You always want to be available to help people, but limit your time when it becomes dysfunctional. Focus on being the positive role model in their lives if you really want to help them, and then leave it up to them. You can offer only so much advice to them. Praying for them is far healthier and productive than enabling them.

Having active role models in your life who project the idea that they can do anything they set their minds to and watching them complete their dreams and goals is pretty amazing. It will have the same effect in your life if you allow it. One of my CrossFit coaches, Jonathan Jorgenson, once told me, "It's what you do with the failure that counts." Think about that. We all make mistakes, have issues, and deal with some negativity here and there, but how we turn those things around into something positive is what makes a difference in your life and in the lives of others. Turning your failures into something successful is one of the requirements that help us reach our goals. Coach Jorgenson's statement was profound and helped me reach my fitness goals.

Poor nutrition choices will definitely cause mental problems and, of course, physical problems, which exacerbate depression. We will address nutrition later in the book multiple times. Your body is an amazing piece of work. You have to keep it well tuned, and that includes the brain. Hormones need to stay in check. Working with holistic or naturopath doctors is highly recommended before embarking on a fitness and nutrition plan. They can teach you to treat areas of concern with naturopathy rather than synthetic drugs, going after the issues and fixing rather than patching for a while with drugs.

Don't get me wrong—drugs have a time and place, and we need to be grateful for that. But way too many people take drugs to treat their conditions rather than make the changes that can cure them, maybe even for life. People make these Band-Aid choices for many different reasons, such as convenience, no discipline, insurance, big pharma, and lack of knowledge, for the most part.

Keeping your hormones balanced and in check gives the mind and body a great place to be in. A simple annual blood test reveals a lot of information that can save your life, not to mention feed you information about how you're taking care of yourself. Deeper testing, called subclinical testing, can provide more information on what state your body is in. Having these types of tests done through urine, blood, saliva, and brain mapping can provide results that will keep you well informed on what is going on inside your body and give you the opportunity to change things for your optimal health. Keeping the data on a spreadsheet makes it easy for you to compare from year to year and also helps keep your doctor organized. It's never too soon to start taking these lab tests for baselines.

You can look for possible changes over time, catch things early, and then make changes to fix them.

I saw a report the other day that one out of three children in the United States has high bad cholesterol, and children should have their first cholesterol check at nine years old and then again in adolescence. I think this is a great opportunity to set them up for a good shot at staying healthy. My husband had the idea to put my lab results on a spreadsheet, so it would be a great way of understanding and reading the labs quickly and seeing any changes. This also helps my doctor organize when I go in once a year. That way, I don't have to sit and watch her fumble through her paper file, trying to find last year's results.

Ask for copies of all your lab work and medical records for your own private file at home. You will never be sorry for doing that, and most doctors appreciate it. It saves so much time and gives you more time with your doctor to ask questions. If your doctor doesn't appreciate the fact that you take charge of your own health and are organized to help both of you, perhaps you need a new doctor.

Managing your stress is important. If you do not manage your stress, it can affect your body just like alcohol or drug abuse. People have many ways of managing their stress. For some, it may take the form of meditating, reading, exercising, or getting a massage weekly. You have to be the one who figures out what works best for you and your situation. When I talk about managing your stress, I am referring to managing it with something healthy. This could be a revelation here, people—ask yourself what you are managing your stress with. Is it comfort food, several glasses of wine each night, or a long walk on a nature trail? With all this being said, dig deep inside, and put on your mental toughness to have the discipline to work through all these things. Have the mental toughness to recognize when stress is coming down the pike, and manage it—or manage it so perfectly, it never arrives!

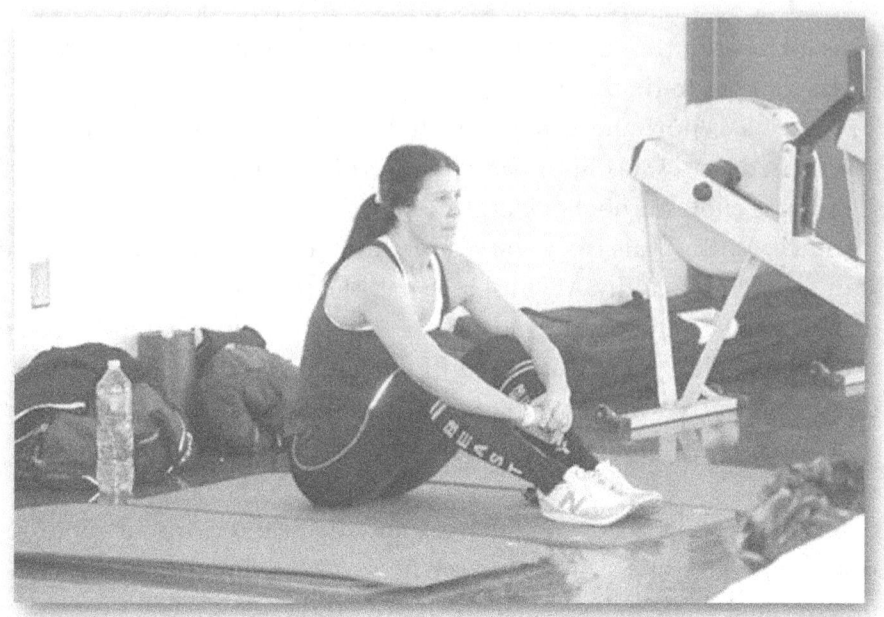

Focused and calm at NorCal Masters competition.

CHAPTER 3

NUTRITION

THIS IS A tough topic, and I want to point out again how important it is to check with your functional medicine, naturopathic, or holistic doctor before change. I believe that the food choices we make are 80 percent of staying healthy. You have to eat to fuel, and what you eat depends on your fuel needs. You want to be eating fresh foods, like organic vegetables, herbs, and fruits. Eating it raw as often as possible will provide the most nutrients. Eating fermented foods is a great way to get your raw food. This type of food is loaded with probiotics which aid in the digestive process. When you cook food, you lose nutrient value. If you chose to cook, cook for the shortest amount of time as possible, and do not use a microwave oven. This will preserve the most nutrient values of your vegetables.

Most of the items in packages or boxes are not real food. If you read the labels, you will see that such foods are filled with chemicals, sugar, and other harmful ingredients that wreak havoc on your body, especially over time. Look up some of the words on the labels sometime, and you will understand why it's way better to eat fresh, whole food. Eat organic, grass-fed beef; wild game; organic chicken; and fresh, wild fish and wild seafood. The *wild* part means "not farmed." Grass-fed and grass-finished beef has the same omega 3-6 ratio that fish has. An animal cannot be grained to hold the correct 3-6 healthy ratios. Once the animal is grained, those numbers change for the worst. *Grass fed* and *grass finished* mean that the animal has not been given any grain.

Eating foods that are high in the good fats, like nuts, coconuts, and avocados, is super nutritious and promotes a higher level of the good cholesterol in our bodies. All those referenced foods should be eaten on a regular basis, with the vegetables being the largest percentage to keep you alkaline. Disease does not like to manifest in an alkaline environment, but it loves the acidic pH, which is created by eating processed foods and too much protein. A great reference book on understanding pH is *Your Health, Your Choice* by Dr. M. Ted Morter. Fresh juicing daily or every other day is an optimal way of getting in some powerful super greens. Smoothies also help you get your veggies in, as well as your super fruits, especially in the Vitamix! It can smooth out the chunkiest vegetable into the prettiest colors; try a beet smoothie sometime.

The Paleo diet is a great plan to follow. A nice book on the subject is *The Paleo Solution* by Robb Wolf. Again, depending on what you are fueling for, you may need to add some foods that are not Paleo. Keeping the protein grams down is wise. Eating too much protein can happen easily on the Paleo diet, and protein produces acid ash. Again, we need to eat fewer acid-producing ash foods and more alkaline-producing foods. Organic produce is a must. Staying away from highly toxic fertilizers, genetically modified organisms (GMOs), and pesticides will increase your chances of staying healthy. Yes, you have to pay a little more, and sometimes the organic produce is limited depending on what part of the country you live in, but it's worth it. You should go ahead and pay extra now, or pay a lot later when you are sick.

This is where growing your own garden can be advantageous in numerous ways. Teaching your children to grow a garden is priceless. Make sure you plant heirloom seeds, which are seeds that have not been genetically modified. Even the smallest spaces are capable of having a garden. It tastes so good, too. I can taste the difference when something is fresh or ripe. Some fruits, veggies, and nuts are protected by a hard skin or shell, which actually won't require you to buy organic because it doesn't make a difference. A list is out there that says organic is a must for these fruits because they are heavily treated with pesticides. Apples and strawberries are two on the list you want to be sure to buy organic. Do your research, and find out the difference.

Here is a website for more information; http://www.mindbodygreen.com/0-17624/12-fruits-veggies-with-the-most-pesticides-2015-dirty-dozen.html

You can get very smart about your food choices. When you pick your produce, select items that are high in antioxidants, high in the good fats, and alkaline-ash producing to help keep your pH level alkaline. If you produce an acidic pH, you are stepping up your game to invite disease in, and you feel yucky. Poor health thrives when pH levels are more acidic. Many books address the topic of pH in the body. I would highly recommend reading one or at least Googling it so you can understand how our pH levels affect our health. Learning how to check your pH is also a smart way of staying on top of your health. Knowing the vegetables and fruits to eat to keep your pH in check is good knowledge. I am warning you in advance, however, that myriad mixed opinions on this topic exist. Picking foods that produce alkaline ash over acid ash is a healthier choice anyway, so depending on what side you take, receiving the benefits of alkaline-producing foods could be twofold.

Where you buy your food is also very important. I know not everyone has the opportunity that I do living on the central coast of California, but try to do your best when shopping. You always want to purchase organic. I started out at the produce section of the regular grocery store, but soon I found that they did not always have what I wanted. I next went to a grocery store or health food store that specialized in foods that are organic or natural. They are more expensive, but the selections are better, and many of it is local—which can mean fresher. I discovered farmers' markets soon after, but I had to be careful because not all the sellers were always selling organic, pesticide-free produce. Sometimes, people will mislead you for the sole purpose of a profit. Get to know your farmers.

The next step I took was actually finding a farm that grew and sold their vegetables and fruit in one place. Now *that's* getting to know your farmers. Besides selling their own produce, they selected a few other farmers and ranchers to bring their products in because they were trustworthy and had good organic product, such as local unpasteurized honey and grass-fed and grass-finished beef. I go to this farm twice a week to purchase 90 percent of my food. There are no middlemen or transportation costs, so it is cost effective for what I am getting. Besides, it was just picked, and now I am eating it. Other than picking it from my own gardens, it doesn't get much better than this. You have to look around, and you can find fresh and healthy. Big-box stores cannot compare on any level, period.

Water is something most of us do not drink enough of, and drinking the correct water can also be difficult. Finding and drinking the purest form of water is always my goal. I also try to drink from glass or metal bottles rather than plastic. Tap water is generally a poor form of water to drink because many chemicals have been intentionally added to it, and then there are the amounts of toxins and chemicals that have been added not so intentionally. I actually cannot even recall the last time I drank a glass of tap water. I turn down tap water even at a restaurant or friend's house. I installed a whole house water filtration system on my home as well as a reverse osmosis unit for drinking water.

The amount of water you need to drink is just like your food amount and type; your circumstances and environments dictate that. The basic rule is half your body weight in ounces. Most people don't drink even a quarter of that, but they ingest lots of other fluids that are not healthy, and they think they are hydrating their bodies. Many health issues are linked with dehydration. I know of young people who went to the ER, only to learn they were dehydrated. Come on, really? Is it that hard to drink water? I guess so, if you drink soda and other sugared drinks. Major health issues come from long bouts of not having proper hydration in our bodies. The bottom line is easy to understand here: most people are not drinking enough good water by any means. Take charge, and be responsible for your own hydration. I have actually heard people say, "I don't like the taste of water." Well, change it up, and put a drop of lime or wild-orange essential oil in it. Squeeze some fresh lemon juice, and add that. Whatever it takes, stay hydrated with good water for your health's sake.

CHAPTER 4

SUPPLEMENTS AND HERBS

EVERYBODY HAS A need for supplements. Figuring out what supplements best work for you individually and taking them provide huge health benefits in so many ways. Everyone should be taking a basic, high-quality vitamin and mineral supplement of some sort. Your doctor can test you to see what you are low in and how you are absorbing your nutrients. Regardless of how careful you are with your food plan, I am pretty sure it is impossible to consume all the vitamins and minerals you require through eating alone. The environment has changed so much that the produce grown has less nutrient value now. Keeping your vitamins and minerals at optimal levels provides healthy, vibrant skin; strong bones; shiny, ample hair; a healthy gut; healthy gums and teeth; thick, fast-growing nails; and lots of energy—just to name a few of the benefits.

I chose to have the benefits rather than being deficient and facing health issues. Vitamin D has come to the front lines of the vitamins. Many claims and studies state that vitamin D promotes the absorption of calcium. Well, that's a no-brainer. You should take it, especially if you are an athlete or concerned about aging. Having lower levels of vitamin D can increase your odds of several types of cancer and diabetes. You may be asking yourself, "How do I know if I'm getting enough vitamin D?" Taking a simple blood test administered by your doctor can give you those answers. I would bet—if you are not taking a vitamin D supplement—that you are very low. You cannot get enough from the sun. Liquid vitamin D drops are an easy way to get your vitamin D levels up and are reasonably priced. Vitamin C is also getting a lot of attention, and higher dosages are becoming mainstream, especially for those wanting to build up their immune systems. Having a strong immune system is crucial in staying healthy.

Once you get past the basic program, you want to look at your specific needs and start addressing those issues. Protein powders are a superb way of getting your protein in easily and quickly. If you are juicing, you can add it to your juice or smoothies. Add it to organic oatmeal. As with everything else, pay attention to your product, and educate yourself on the different types of proteins available. Quality is a priority. Protein powder and protein bars are easy to travel with and convenient snacks to carry around in your purse or gym bag. Having prepared enough to have this handy can protect you from eating junk or overeating when your schedule gets out of whack. Just make sure you read the labels and understand the ingredients. A lot of junk is loaded with sugar, synthetic sweetener, fillers, thickeners, and grains. Synthetic sweeteners are everywhere, and they have been linked to making people very sick. Here is an example article from Dr. Mercola's website in reference to artificial sweeteners: http://articles.mercola.com/sites/articles/archive/2016/03/30/artificial-sweeteners-cause-cancer.aspx. If you are an athlete, it may be difficult at times to get your required grams of protein through home-cooked meals, so adding a protein powder once or twice a day can help you meet your daily needs. Even vegan protein powders are available. I do think you ought to be careful with the amount of protein you're taking in; many people are taking in too much for their bodies to utilize. Ideally, one-half gram of protein per pound of lean body mass weight is a good measure. Eating too much protein can cause a decline in health, including high blood sugar, weight gain, and kidney stones. Other health issues include creating acid pH, as I mentioned before.

Another supplement that is getting a lot of attention because of its many benefits is fish oil. You could eat a lot of fatty fish to gain your benefits from fish oil, but then you may have a mercury issue to deal with. Fish oil will help you maintain an already-healthy blood-cholesterol profile. It appears to raise the good-cholesterol ratios of HDL (high-density lipoprotein cholesterol) to LDL (low-density lipoprotein choles-terol) in the body when they are already in a healthy range. Studies have shown that when you take in higher levels of fatty acids, like fish oils, you support healthy bones. It also reduces pain and swelling. Mood support is another benefit of fish oil. Research has indicated that if you take fish oil in your diet daily, it can offer mood support by naturally supporting your serotonin level, which is the "feel good" hormone.

Carbs also do just that. We eat carbs, and they make us feel relaxed and peaceful. We crave them when we are stressed because we know we can get that peaceful feeling from them. We know that those types of carbs are not good for us. Promoting that feel-good hormone through fish oil is a better choice. It has to be a good-quality fish oil, not whatever is popular at the time at the local gym. Do your research, please.

You can also receive fatty acids in a vegetarian form and avoid the possibility of mercury altogether. It's the eicosapentaenoic acid (EPA)/docosahexaenoic acid (DHA), fatty acids that you are after. Again, you have to be responsible for your supplement picks. Don't rely on what others are saying or doing. Understanding what you are putting into your body not only is a no-brainer, but it makes it easier to explain when someone asks you why you are taking the fish oil and why you chose the more costly brand. You want to be able to understand and explain to others what you are doing. That could lead to helping some-one else.

The supplement list goes on and on. So many are out there that help each and every one of us in so many different ways. Once you get past the basic program of vitamins and minerals, you can write your own prescription for yourself by doing your own research and identifying what your own personal needs are at the time. I say "at the time" because it will change depending on what you are doing. Also, new research is always bringing in new findings. Your health may change, and you may need something added, or maybe you will need to remove something. Once your research is complete and you know what you need, you verify that with your doctor. Supplements can be a great alternative to some drug prescriptions. That can be tricky, though. If you are fortunate enough to have insurance, the insurance company isn't going to pay for your supplements and vitamins, but it will cover your drug prescriptions. You have to decide again: pay more now, or pay more later? Paying more later can mean paying more than just money. Preventative measures are worth every dime.

CHAPTER 5

DETOX

DETOXING IS IMPORTANT, especially in the environment we are living in nowadays with so many harmful chemicals and pollution. We are exposed to over seven hundred chemicals and metals per day. These chemicals are in the beds we sleep on, our food, our water, and even our air we breathe. People are eating large amounts of sugars and grains in the form of processed foods, which are loaded with chemicals. You probably won't be familiar with most of the ingredients on the labels. The chemicals are used as preservatives, thickeners, and more. Look them up sometime. I'm sure you will cringe once you learn what the chemicals are and what they do to our bodies. We can take only so much before we start breaking down with diseases. We want to achieve optimal health so that we can thrive and be our best in life. Being toxic can make normal, everyday living difficult.

Detoxing is a cleaning of the blood. Our bodies do that by removing toxins from the blood in the liver; there, they are eliminated. Our bodies also get rid of toxins through our other organs, too, like our lungs, kidneys, lymph nodes, intestines, and skin. Our skin is our largest organ. What you put on it, such a lotions and sunscreens, goes right through the skin. When these toxins are not properly filtered out, every cell in our bodies becomes compromised. Once compromised, they become weak, and bad things start to happen. Most of us are now in a mode of toxic overload, and some of it we cannot control, like the air we breathe. However, we can help our bodies bring the toxin levels out.

There are lots of methods or recipes for detoxing. You can do a cleansing detox for a week through a juice fast, for example. But I think you should work on your daily detox by eating properly to begin with, then detoxing. It's not going to do you much good to do a ten-day cleanse if you start eating poorly again.

We already discussed eating real, fresh food and a good, hearty diet made up mostly of organic veggies and fruits. Eat small amounts of organic nuts and seeds. Eat organic meats and wild fish. Drink plenty of pure water. Not only is preparing your own meals as often as possible less expensive, but you also know what you are eating, for the most part. Stay away from food in boxes and packages. Those items aren't fresh and usually aren't real, whole food.

Another form of detoxing is sweating. You can achieve that through exercise or a sauna—ideally, both. It's important to shower off the sweat directly after exercising or taking a sauna. You have just sweated out the toxins, so don't let those reabsorb into your pores. Actually, scrubbing with a sea sponge will help eliminate those toxins even better while you're showering or bathing. Being able to exercise and visit the sauna is ideal. We definitely need to be working out, but sometimes we can't because of certain work schedules, traveling, or other obligations. That's when a sauna comes in handy. Infrared would be my choice. Having one installed in your garage, backyard, or home would make things easy and relaxing. They are quite popular now, so you can go to certain clubs and pay to use one as well. Many gyms also have saunas, which are great to hop in after a workout. Using essential oils in the saunas will aid in detoxing, and that's an extra bonus.

Speaking of essential oils, you can use them in different ways to detox, such as diffusing them in the air or using them in your bathwater or shower to massage them into your skin. One specific oil that comes to mind is lemongrass, but many others are available if you don't like its scent. Soaping up with an activated charcoal soap pulls toxins from the skin while bathing.

You can take many different supplements to help you detox, as well as greens and super fruits. Milk thistle is a great herb to detox with after surgery. It helps remove the anesthesia out through the liver more efficiently.

Much can be said for detoxing. If you work in an environment where you are exposed to chemicals and gases, you better be detoxing. You will feel so much better, and your body will function more efficiently. You can take tests to find out how toxic you are and what type of toxicity is in your body if you want to be more specific. This is really the safest way to detox. Find a functional-medicine doctor in your area, and have him or her run a series of tests on you to find out where your overloads are. Then, set forth with them on your own protocol.

Detoxing can be dangerous, so it is best to talk with a professional who has a lot of knowledge in this area. Preparing yourself to detox is wise, and the physician can explain how that's done best for you. The tests are costly and most likely not covered by your health insurance. But your life is worth it. Make it a priority. Detoxing is crucial in today's age to stay healthy. Our children should also be detoxing.

CHAPTER 6

STAYING ACTIVE AND EXERCISING

WE TALKED ABOUT my childhood and how fortunate I was to be exposed to lots of activity early on. I think there is definitely a lot of hype going on regarding exercise, and people are trying to become fit or fitter in addition to learning to eat better. Then there is this current generation of kids, hunched over playing video games, texting, and participating in social media for hours on end all while eating large quantities of unhealthy food. I saw a study on Dr. Mercola's website the other day that states that the average child today is spending nine of every twenty-four hours on social media (http://articles. mercola.com/sites/articles/archive/2015/12/16/teens-media-usage. aspx). What? I know there are some positive things coming out of all that technology, and I enjoy it myself daily. On the other hand, there is definitely negativity that comes out of it. The poor posture that comes from hunching over the devices leads to internal rotation of the shoulders, and this leads to other health issues. The inactivity unfortunately replaces time that could be utilized being active through so many different ways. I wish parents would help their children find a better balance with smartphones and other devices. I see a lot of parents hand their phones over to their children to keep them entertained, which makes my heart so sad. How about give them a little workout, and then they might want to take a nap or even go to bed earlier? Maybe have them help you learn a new recipe that is healthy. Start teaching them how to cook when they are young and still heavily influenced by you.

Getting some exercise daily can be a challenge for some and easy peasy for others. Something is out there for every person, regardless of age, experience, handicaps, or current state of fitness. There is an endless supply of advice, information, and teaching on exercise. But ultimately, we are responsible for our own fitness. Find out what works best for you, and stick with it.

I myself am more of a competitive athlete and have a bachelor's of science in teaching physical education and five CrossFit certifications. There isn't much I have not taught, tried, or competed in. I spent a lot of time competing in skiing, cycling, running, bodybuilding, powerlifting, softball, triathlons, and barrel racing.

I actually had a shot at cycling at one point while living in Alaska. I was ranked as one of the top female cyclists in Alaska and was invited to train at the Olympic training center to be a possible contender for the US Women's Cycling Team. After arriving at the Olympic training center in Colorado Springs, I was sent home shortly thereafter by the head coach, not for lack of athletic ability or discipline in the training but for discovering that I was pregnant. One morning I was not feeling well. The head coach took me to a clinic where they performed a pregnancy test. The results were positive. I was told to go home, have an abortion, and come back. I discussed this with my dad when I arrived home because he had supported me in getting me to the training center and had so much hope in me. I was disappointed in myself for disappointing him. Dad was my idol. I loved him dearly and wanted nothing more than to please him. I told him what they said, and we both looked at each other and knew what the right choice was. Gabrieal Monroe Ann Budke was born two weeks early, on my dad's birthday. Dad said it was the best birthday present he was ever given. It truly was and still is the best thing he has ever said to me. I will never forget that day.

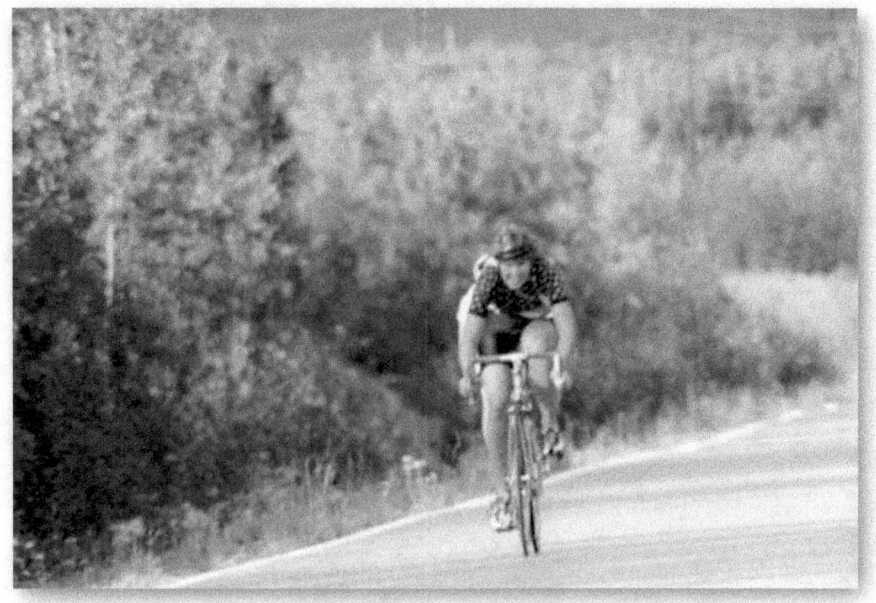

Road racing in Alaska.

I also skied on a cross-country ski scholarship for the University of Alaska at Anchorage. I didn't have much experience because I had focused on being a competitive downhill skier, yet I was recruited because of my cycling quadriceps and hamstring development. The assistant coach at UAA at the time came to me and asked if I would go out and hit the courses with him to see if I could make the traveling team. I made the team that day, to my surprise. It brought me lots of opportunities and good times. The same coach who sought after me for a cross-country ski scholarship also exposed me to triathlons, where I placed on every podium. I had tons of sports and sport competitions throughout my whole life thereafter. I figured out if I had a clean diet and stayed consistent in my training, I could excel at any sport.

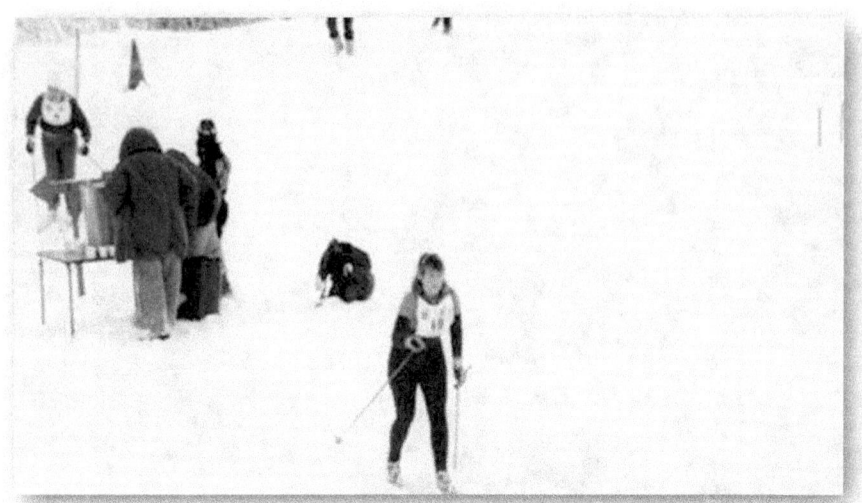

Competing for University of Alaska in Lake Placid, New York

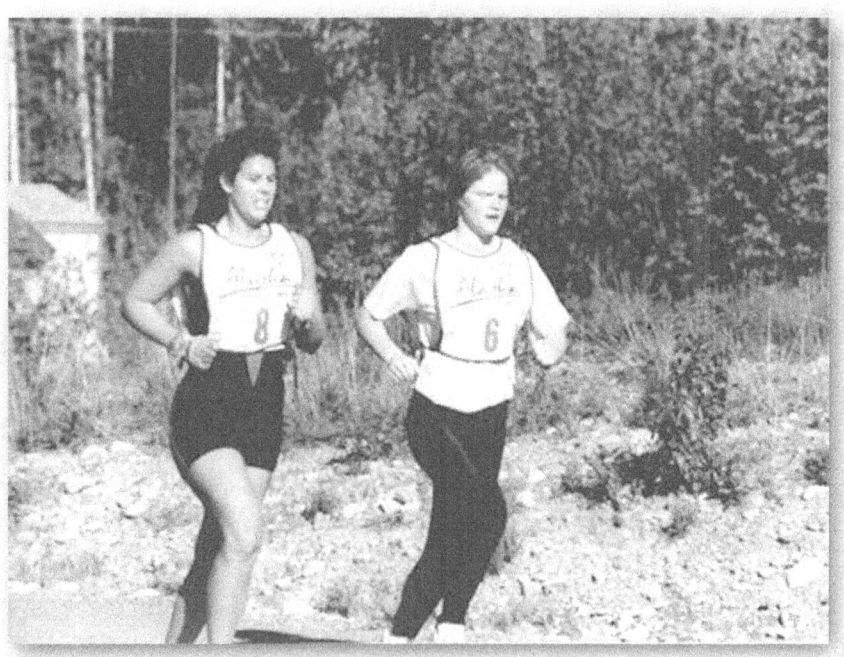

Triathlon in Alaska.

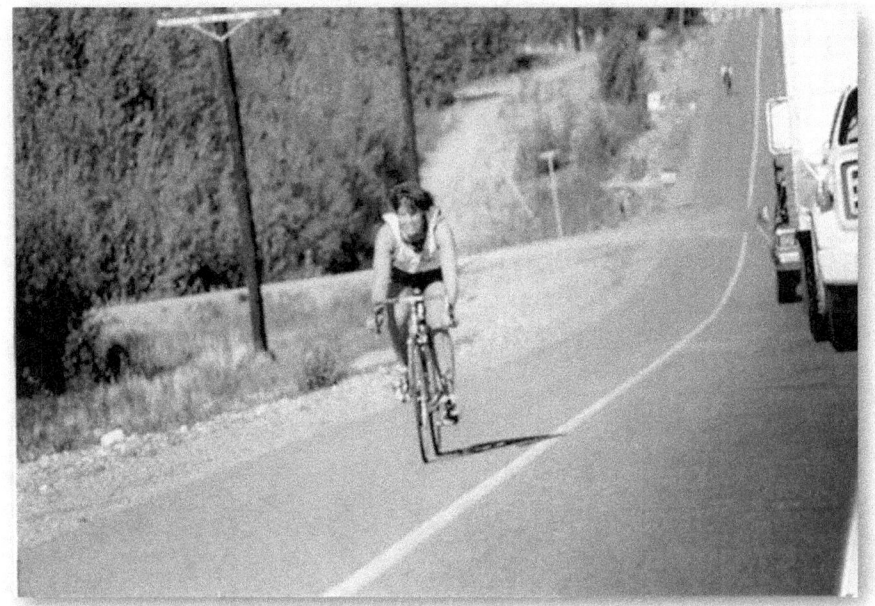

Cycling stage of triathlon.

Once I graduated from UAA, I found a way to stay fit and eat healthy through competitive bodybuilding. After doing three successful bodybuilding shows, I jumped into powerlifting and reached a national competitive level, where I broke records and took second in my weight class at the age of thirty-six. Powerlifting is a sport where you lift as heavy as you can in your weight class and are scored on the total number for three lifts: the bench press, dead lift, and back squat. I found out that hard work and discipline paid off again.

Even when I was not training for something competitive, I always worked on keeping my body in shape and tried to eat as healthy as possible. I would lift weights, take dance classes, teach aerobics, swim laps, run, and ride horses. Staying fit and eating heathy was not always easy, especially while living in Alaska. As I aged into my forties, the body fat was creeping in. I had to start pressing in and studying my whole body to find out what I was lacking. I had to find professionals to help me design a complete program that my body needed. Moving from Alaska to California was by far the biggest help. Exercising outdoors in the sun and having fresh food available to me for a fraction of the price was awesome. I had started competing in barrel racing on horseback in Alaska. The season in Alaska was short; however, in California, the season is twelve months of the year. I was in heaven in California. I was home.

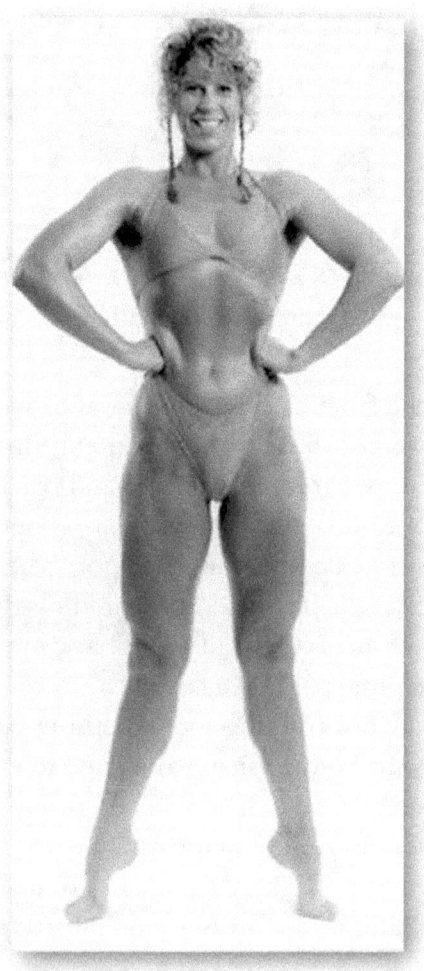

First body building competition – placed fourth.

Speaking of heaven, when I entered the field of barrel racing in Alaska, I was confident in my Christianity. I took a huge leap of faith and started evangelizing in the field of barrel racing. I was able to carry that momentum forward in California. I competed in many different organizations and circuits. I was on the road year round competing in most of the western states, wearing God on my sleeve.

When I was competing in barrel racing in my early fifties, I applied like a crazy women to compete in a bikini barrel race. Insane, right? I thought my husband was going to come unglued when I told him. Barrel racing is crazy enough on its own, but add wearing only a bikini, and that changes things up.

Barrel racing is when you take a fast horse and run around a cloverleaf pattern for time. I envisioned my bikini top popping off as I flew around a turn. Yet my husband chose to support me rather than fight me. I was working very hard at the time to stay fit by taking spin classes and lifting weights but believed I needed an additional edge to compete against the eleven other selected woman, who I knew would be much younger than me by twenty or thirty years. In my mind, they would have perfectly young bikini bodies with possible enhancements. Plus, they would be some of the best riders on the fastest horses.

I had been hearing about this newer sport called CrossFit, so I thought I would give that a go. When I approached the CrossFit box about my goals, they were obliged to take me on as an athlete. The thing that sold me on trying CrossFit was that no two workouts are the same. The workouts are programmed new each day and written on a whiteboard. I was thinking that it would be amazing to keep my body guessing and responding uniquely at every workout. It would definitely be interesting, to say the least. No more monotonous and boring workouts!

I think it's important to take you through this outstanding journey I have been on simply by stumbling on to CrossFit, trying something new to get fitter, and following my heart to always improve myself. I want to share with you how I became the fittest I have ever been at age fifty-five and how CrossFit carries over into so much more in your life and community. You never know what plans God has for you, so listen and act when he speaks.

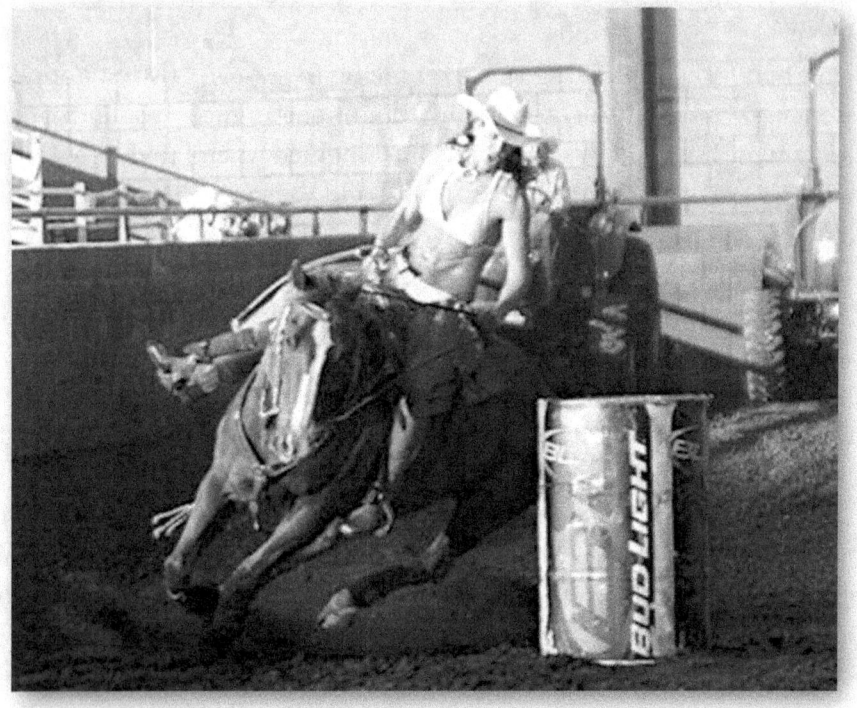

My first and only bikini barrel race at age 53.

I found my first few days at CrossFit absolutely amazing, and I was hooked right off the bat. I want to describe CrossFit to those of you who have not tried it or do not understand it. The building or place where you work out is called a box rather than a gym. All are individually owned; to advertise the CrossFit name, they must be an affiliate of CrossFit. It's similar to purchasing a franchise. They pay an annual fee to use the CrossFit name. The owner and the employed coaches must follow rules and regulations to become and stay an affiliate. They are required to have a CrossFit level-one certification, which requires special CrossFit training. This means their athlete members will be provided with the best training possible, ensuring good form, technique, and safety.

Generally speaking, the box will be located in a warehouse-style building providing lots of high ceiling space and plenty of room to perform the hundreds of different functional moves. Equipment ranges from barbells to tires! It's functional fitness at its best, all performed in an hour or less from a warm-up to a cool down, usually designed to increase your range of motion (ROM). Functional fitness consists of performing moves that you would do in everyday life, such as picking something up off the ground in proper form, avoiding injury, and maybe even saving someone's life. No two workouts are ever the same. How cool is that? A workout of the day (WOD) is always surprising your body and mind. No more routines, and your body is going to respond far better because it has nothing to get used to. It's pretty ingenious, in my opinion. Several CrossFit WODs are named after people or events. For example, the Hero WODs are named after heroes from the military and first responders who have all passed away in the line of duty. Another category example is called the Benchmark Girls, such as Cindy or Amanda. These WODs are designed to be both challenging and fun but can also be scaled down to accommodate anyone.

Classes usually start very early in the morning and end later in the evening, giving people with almost any work schedule an opportunity to join in. Most of the larger boxes provide day care, too. Many of the boxes will have an open gym time for those who want to come in and do extra work. Those are usually the athletes who desire to compete or athletes who want to conquer certain moves or skills that require extra work. Saturdays are usually a day where the box has one free class, when anyone can come in and join to get a feel for what CrossFit is. There's also the option of dropping in if you are traveling, which can be free, or having a drop-in fee. Many times the fee is waived if you buy a T-shirt.

Depending on the class size, at least one certified instructor is on the floor, ready to instruct and assist. He or she is always focusing on safety and technique. Before members can step into a class, they are required to take on-ramp classes, which move them through a one-on-one or small ratio of coach-to-member instruction of the basic fundamentals of CrossFit. These classes usually last an hour or less and run for approximately two weeks. While attending the on-ramp sessions, the new members will also have opportunities to learn about diet and mobility, two important items that will improve fitness gains and help keep injury at bay. Once members have finished the course, they are ready to enter into a CrossFit class with basic CrossFit skills under their belts, giving them confidence and reducing the risk of injury. Once they enter into classes, the attending coach will assist and remind them of the basic fundamentals while they learn new skills.

As the person behind designing the workouts, the programmer can design his or her own programming or subscribe to some of the very successful boxes or independent programmers who offer up their programming to the general public, sometimes for a fee. The programmer puts a lot of thought into these workouts, which focus on strength, skills, endurance, agility, and intensity. You may notice in the programing that certain time frames are used for certain movements, usually progressing along in a six-week cycle or longer. I enjoy the boxes that use a program method over time, which allows the athletes time to improve and see their hard work and effort pay off with great results.

I was surprised at how simple CrossFit boxes are. No fancy, high-dollar equipment to speak of. No weight machines all lined up, covering all the floor space from wall to wall. No fancy locker rooms, tanning beds, or smoothie bars. Barbells, kettlebells, rowers, and wall balls were the first pieces of equipment I noticed and quickly became fond of. When I mingled with the members, I was amazed at all the different walks of life and ages who were "WODing" right next to me. On one side of me was a police officer, and on the other side was a college student. The environment was positive, uplifting, and friendly. I fit in right from the start because of the many different mixes of personalities, and everyone seemed so focused and happy to be there.

CrossFit combines weight lifting, gymnastics, and agility. Anybody can do it because you can scale a movement to meet your ability level. Scaling is also a benefit for someone injured or handicapped. Many of the movements may be scaled to reach an athlete's current status of mobility. Scaling means changing the movement prescribed to make it capable of being performed at a doable method or maybe performing one step of the movement but still focusing on the prescribed movement and muscle group. As you are able to perform each scaled version of the more advanced move, eventually you will master the advanced move. Seeing this happen in other athletes and even myself with many of the movements is self-empowering.

I moved up the ranks of CrossFit rapidly, especially considering my age. The coaches were amazed and said I had enough potential to make it to the CrossFit Games. I had no idea what they were talking about.

I found out what they were talking about rather quickly because they would not let up on my potential and wanted me to commit to a competitive-training class to prepare for the open, which would qualify me for the CrossFit Games. I was focused on getting super lean and jockey-weight light so I could win this bikini barrel race, or at least be the best I could be on the day of the race. I was also conscious about what my body looked like in a skimpy bikini while I galloped my horse as fast she could run. I had to persuade the coaches to help me with this goal first, and then I would turn myself over after the eleven weeks. Then they could put me through their competitive-training methods if they still wanted to. They agreed to my timing. I was thankful for that because the pressure was off for the games for a bit.

Now they had a choice. They could have turned me away if I wasn't going to abide with their program. I made it through the on-ramp program without any issues, and off I went into their classes. They were fun and interesting, and I never encountered a dull moment with all those different moves and different personalities. Immediately in my first class, I realized that my competiveness had not backed down any, even at my mature age. I was quickly trying to finish the work WODs faster than an eighteen-year-old.

When I had committed myself to the eleven weeks to prepare my body for a bikini barrel race on horseback, I had no clue about the venture I was about to embark on. God never ceases to amaze me, and I could hear and see his calling in all things CrossFit, with the windows wide open. I had been ministering in the barrel racing world by opening events in prayer, counseling couples and individuals, and leading people to Christ. It was hard to leave that field to be plopped into a field of new people and a new sport to represent Christ. But I could see his hand in it, and I had to be wide open to his invitation through obedience. The box that a friend had steered me to became my home away from home. This particular box had been open for only a few months. The building was in a good location and had plenty of space because it was quite large and in excellent shape. Because it was a new box, class attendance was small, which provided more individualized attention and more floor space. The owners had made a nice investment in the equipment initially for a startup. There was variety, and everything was new. I was able to reap the benefits that come with a brand-new box.

Once I got through the bikini barrel race, I honored my word to those coaches. I put forth the effort to see if I had what it took to qualify for the 2013 CrossFit Games in the early-fifties-female age category.

I pretty much did what I was told. My first CrossFit coach, Rich, actually commented on several occasions that I was very coachable, and he liked that about me. That's a desirable skill to have as an athlete, but I had no clue what I was doing in CrossFit. I was simply following directions and again honoring my word. I want to emphasize how I feel about that. Throughout my life, I see people sign up for nutritional advice and plans, personal training, and therapy. They are getting all this wonderful paid advice but not following it. It seems to be the trend. I wonder. Is the failure due to where the advice is coming from, or is it on the individual receiving the advice? Are people doing their best? For me, I was doing my best. I was being respectful, honoring my word, and doing my best on the box floor as an athlete. Once you are committed to a goal or your word, no other routes remain. It perplexes me as I try to understand others' choices.

One of the other things that Coach Rich told me in the beginning was that it was important to try to stay independent as a CrossFitter. What did that mean to him? Try to start thinking for yourself. Some examples of this include learning to add your own weights and checking your math twice. Stop asking your coaches the same questions over and over, such as, "How much do you think I should go up in weight today?" In the beginning of learning to CrossFit, those questions make sense, but you have got to be able to learn and take charge of your own workout and stop relying on coaches for every little thing. You are inside your body, and you should be able to feel and decide if you should go up in weight at that moment. It does take practice and knowledge to know and understand those decisions. But to get there, the earlier you start, the quicker you will obtain that skill rather than depending on someone else to give you the answer. Think for yourself; you know yourself better than anybody does. Coach Rich was very adamant about this with me. I am, for the most part, independent, so his rule made sense to me, and you will see it pay off later in a big way. But I have seen others struggle with this. It drives some of the coaches crazy.

I am a hard worker, too, and very competitive. It was the norm for me to give it all I had during every workout. It wasn't long before I could see that I was one of the fittest and fastest athletes in there, regardless of sex or age. This did not make much sense to me, as I did not expect to be so fit and driven in my fifties. This drove me to work smarter and harder. It was fun to meet all these new people and learn about them and what was going on in their lives. Just taking the time to bond with them and learn about them and their families made me realize how much I love people still, and they all had something they needed prayer for. The membership base in this box was predominantly young. Only two other members were older than me, and I had the privilege of working out with one of them.

We quickly became best friends. We had a lot of fun together, and he was positive and funny. I often threatened him that I was going to write a book about some of the funniest things he said and did in there. I knew the book would be a best-seller because I had never laughed so hard.

CrossFit is unique in the sense that the members support one another far deeper than I have ever seen, including in the churches I have grown up in and belonged to. Usually, you don't put your equipment away until the last person is finished. Many will gather around after they have finished their workout and stand by the last athlete, cheering him or her on. We cheer for one another all while competing against ourselves and others. If someone gets hurt, everyone stops his or her workout and attends or supports the injured athlete. Many times, the CrossFit box will attend a Sunday function, such as a hike up a waterfall, and show up with family and friends. They will hold fund-raisers of all shapes and sizes to support one of their own or maybe someone in the community. CrossFit people have often been accused of being a cult because the brotherhood/sisterhood is so strong. It's unique, and I enjoy feeling I'm a part of something like this so soon after joining. CrossFitters have one another's backs.

I had not been training very long when I noticed a local competition coming up, and I asked my coach if I should enter. "Sure," he said. I knew I would not do well because the competition organizers did not have a master's category, which meant I would compete against twenty-year-olds. But I thought it would be a good experience for me to check out CrossFit competition style. I think the competition had about twenty-eight young girls, and I came in twenty-first place and was definitely the oldest. My coach and his family came and coached and supported me, which was great. I was the only one who competed from our box in this local competition. Also, my young nephew, Steven, was staying with me for a year and was trying CrossFit. He was doing really well. He came and supported me and took some terrific pictures with our nice Canon camera. It was cool to look at those photos of me starting in a new sport, and the actual experience was humbling. I learned a lot that day and had a ton of positive reinforcement. One of the owners, who coaches at

Northstate CrossFit, was my judge that day in the lifting portion, and she stated how strong I was naturally. These CrossFit people are special, uplifting, and supportive. I had drunk the Kool-Aid at that point—hook, line, and sinker. Drinking the Kool-Aid is a term CrossFitters use when people allow CrossFit to become a habit in their lives.

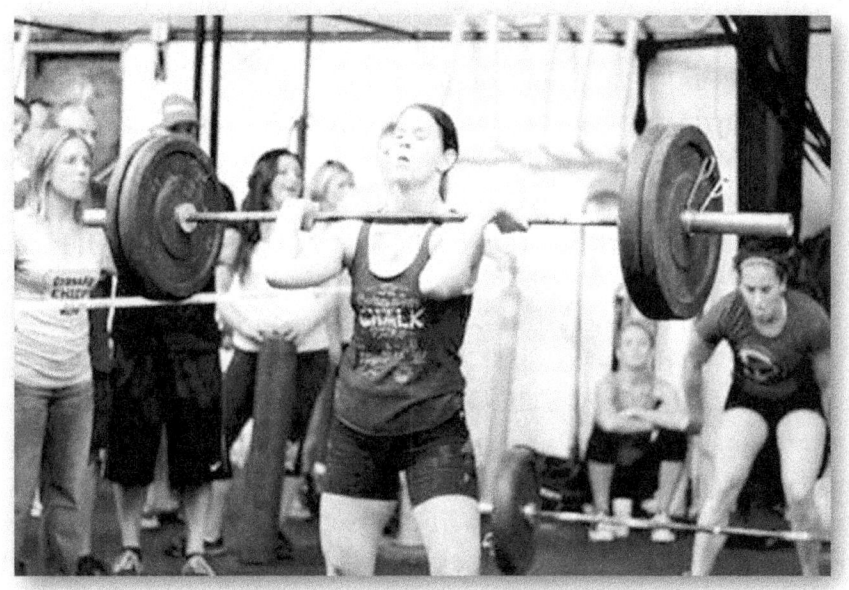

My first CrossFit competition in 2012, "Northstates Fittest "held at Northstate CrossFit.

I discovered another not-so-local competition coming up in San Francisco. It was the biggest competition and as close to competing at the CrossFit Games you could get for masters in CrossFit. It's called the NorCal Masters. I was beyond myself with excitement. I highly recommend this competition for any master who wants to go to the games or any master who wants to compete in his or her own age group. It can help you season yourself for the games. The competition WODs are very similar to those at the games. The judges are superb. You will be competing against masters who have been to the games at least once or many times. Some might be about to qualify for the games for their first time. The age groups are separated by five years, starting with forty-year-olds, which is just like in the games. Many competitions group you into an over-forty group. That's tough because you could be fifty-seven and competing against a forty-year-old.

The venue is amazing and has a ton of windows that overlook San Francisco Bay. The equipment is top notch, and some of it is innovative. The prizes make it worth the travel time and money. Plenty of vendors are available with quality equipment and healthy food choices. The competition organizers limit the number of entries in each age bracket so that the competition does not run well into the night. I have noticed over the years that a lot of masters put it off because they think it's too close to the open CrossFit competition, as it is in the middle of January. The open is the first official CrossFit competition on the road to qualifying for the games. This is usually held in late March. I highly disagree with this type of thinking; compared to the games, this is the best experience from a competition for a master on the West Coast. The organizers do a professional job running this show—first class all the way. It's a great opportunity to prepare for the games, and it's also a great chance for a master to compete at a higher level and in his or her age bracket. It could be the only chance of competing at a higher level if you never qualify for the games. I cannot say enough good things about the NorCal Masters and the owners of the show—T. J. and his wife, Allison. Allison has also written a book about CrossFit, The Power of Community. I bought it, read it, and passed it on.

I found out at this competition what it's like to be an independent athlete. Coach Rich and his family came to support Rich's dad, who was also competing and me. His dad had an accident early in the show, which caused the whole family to depart to the nearest hospital to comfort and be with him. After he was released, the family got the flu, and they were tucked away in their hotel or driving home the entire time I was competing for two days. Rich's dad actually broke his collar bone, which required surgery. He healed from that and went to the games again in 2014. He was a good example of overcoming an injury both physically and mentally by doing his recovery correctly. I'm proud of that man.

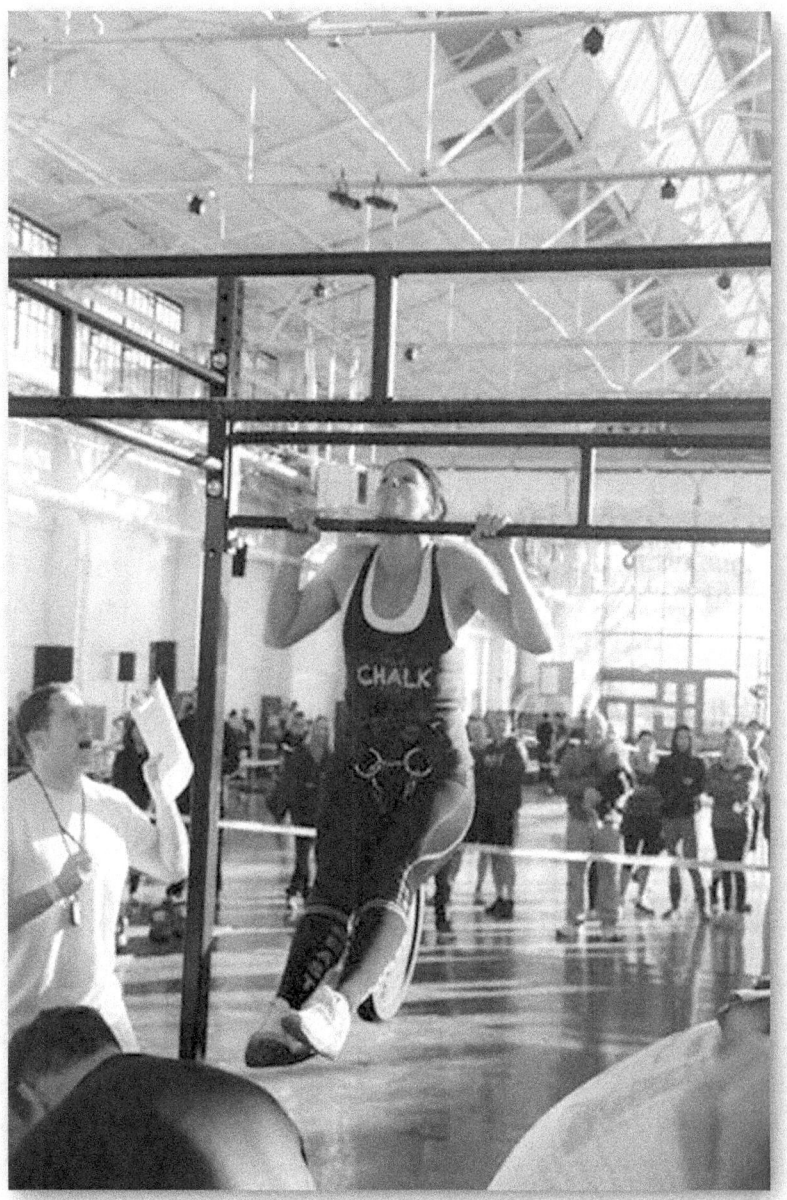

Weighted pullups at the NorCal Masters, my second competition.

I think being at this competition without my coach's support wasn't much of a challenge for me. He had embedded in me early on that I shouldn't rely on him, and I never did. That tip paid off well. I did great and placed fourth out of twenty women in my age group. Several of those women had been to the games many times. They were tough and prepared, and I was the best I could be at the time. This was my second CrossFit competition, and it was actually quite fun. It gave me a good idea of how I was stacking up against other CrossFit women who competed in my age group. Maybe I would do well in the upcoming open CrossFit competition.

I was fortunate to have a primary coach who understood how valuable I was to have never sustained a major injury. He told me numerous times to focus on remaining uninjured. I thought he was protective of me on that issue, and I now know how important that was and is. That would become pivotal in my CrossFit world-level competitive career.

Within the first year of training CrossFit, I qualified to attend my first CrossFit Games in Los Angeles in 2013. To qualify to compete in the CrossFit Games, I had to compete in the open. This was a five-week competition held in the individual boxes with a certified judge onboard. The scores are submitted to CrossFit headquarters once a week. In my age group, they would take the top twenty women from around the world who competed in the open. At fifty-three years of age, I came in seventeenth place. As I was going through the open, it did not dawn on me that this could happen until I was in week four. I was scrolling through the results, and I thought, "I really can do this." They were right.

Boy, did that change up the pressure. Suddenly, things were not so fun. I allowed myself to feel a ton of pressure. One of the ways I chose to deal with it was by allowing myself to find a couple to pray for me as I was finishing the open. The open was grueling for me because I was such a rookie. I had to repeat all the WODs except one. I felt alone inside, as if no one could relate to what was going on with me. If you've done the open and dealt with Dave Castro's hardcore programming, you know how much fun it is to repeat WODs to obtain a better score, only to wear yourself out for the next week's competition. So, I put my little prayer team together with Royce and Tara. Before I had to repeat my last and hardest WOD, I had one of my crazy dreams. The WOD was thrusters and chest-to-bar pull-ups (C2B) in as many rounds as possible (AMRAP). If you know CrossFit, you know how painful these two can be together. I shared the dream with Tara and Royce, whom I had asked to pray for me. I was being pummeled with fireballs in my muscle groups that would require me to do C2B, which are advanced body-weight pull-up movements that I could barely perform all while a cloud was over me. I associated the fireballs with fire being added into those muscles, but the cloud confused me. I asked God about the cloud, and He said, "It's me! I have you covered!" So, I knew I was going to do fine. I went into that WOD for the second time with confidence, and my score improved enough to get me to the games.

After the open was finished, I thought I was a fairly consistent athlete, and that's more than likely what was getting me to the games. But my current affiliate coach never addressed my weaknesses after the open. I knew I could do better than this with the right individualized, specialized coaching. After bringing at least one of my weaknesses to my affiliate coach and not getting much of a response, I knew I had to take the initiative on my own to gain improvement if I wanted to become more efficient in the movements at a competitive level. I kept recalling what he had said about not depending on him because he would not always be viable for me. This was one of those times. I had to stay independent.

So, I took it upon myself to research who would be the best coach for me in this particular situation. After much time spent studying coaches around the area, I picked a coach who was experienced in CrossFit; had earned a bachelor's of science degree in exercise science and kinesiology; had competed three times and was on his way to a fourth at a regional level in CrossFit; owned a successful CrossFit box with numerous certs; had previous fitness training and coaching experience before CrossFit; understood and specialized in several of my weak areas; and put God, family, and his business in that order in his life. I had struck a goldmine of help! The icing on the cake was that we hit it off. To this day, I truly adore and love this man as if he's part of my own family. His parents did an amazing job raising him, and I can't say enough about this guy. My husband took a special interest in him as well, and that doesn't happen much, because the love of my life pretty much keeps to himself. Double blessings! I started taking Olympic lifting (OLY) sessions with Jonathan Jorgenson from Northstate CrossFit as I was finishing the open.

I want to stress something right now. We have to take things into our own hands. We have to be responsible for our own nutrition, our own fitness, our own training methods, and our own health. We can't rely on and then blame others for our own choices. The sooner we become responsible for our own choices, the sooner we will succeed. I practice this, and people will hear me say it repeatedly. If you are relying on others for your own success, you could be setting yourself up for failure. What works for me usually does not work for you. We are all different. If things are not working out for you, take charge, and find out what does. That is how you get there. It's a process.

Once I set up this extra training with an additional coach, everything started to change for me. I suddenly realized that I had gotten myself into a huge challenge, and time was of the essence. I was training for the CrossFit Games 2013, and I hardly knew what I was doing in CrossFit. I had only about three months of training time left before the games would start. That's not a lot of time, especially since I had just started CrossFit. The only thing that was popping out in my brain was to work on my OLY. I had no experience in that field and found it to be quite technical, which challenged my brain. I needed to get around to different local boxes to WOD more than once per day to get ready for the games, but my primary coach hadn't suggested this or encouraged me at that point. I basically trained with my primary coach, his father (who had been to the games), and a few others who were considered more of the elite-athlete status. I maintained private lessons with my OLY coach two days per week.

Getting private OLY lessons paid off. Within the first two weeks of technical lessons, I squat snatched in a hang position over one hundred pounds, which was three personal records (PRs) in one: getting one hundred pounds over my head and squat snatching and hang snatching all in one lift. In earlier weeks, I had failed getting one hundred pounds over my head in the open competition several times—not because of strength but because of technique. It was amazing for a fifty-three-year-old woman with no prior OLY lifting to redeem herself in two short weeks. I'm sure my new OLY coach, Jon, was thrilled about this. It is important to take a failure, learn from, and turn it around to something positive.

My problem was that I had no idea how to get underneath the weight bar quickly to receive the weight safely. I knew it was not about the strength but the technique, so it had to be fixed right away to avoid injuries and to move forward as an elite athlete. My OLY coach and I worked diligently on this lift. It did not come easy for me by any means. I had a lot of trouble putting all the parts together. Coach Jon was patient with me, lesson after lesson, right up to the games. He never showed any impatience or frustration with me, which further assured me he was the right guy for this job and all the next jobs. You have to take those types of good qualities into consideration when you are working with someone like this. I don't care how nice or popular they are; they need to be proficient in all the fields needed and of fair market price. They are coaching because they want to help people, are trained upright in it, and can communicate to most people in many different ways. After all, we don't receive communications the same ways. Coach Jon has all that. I was fortunate to have studied and selected the right guy first time out. What a blessing!

Before the open competition, it became apparent to me that it would be in my best interest to get my level-one certification from CrossFit headquarters. I went to Reno and did just that within my first year. That paid off. I got a ton of one-on-one coaching in all the movements, met a ton of big-time CrossFitters and instructors, learned more about training for competitions, passed my exam, earned my certification, and made a lot of connections. It was very expensive to take that course, but it was worth it. I decided to obtain another certification in powerlifting, and that is where I met the amazing A. J. Roberts. He had and may still hold world records in powerlifting. He was the instructor for that course that was also in Reno. Again, I met another group of amazing CrossFit people—some big-time athletes and master-games competitors. I felt special at this clinic because many people were saying nice things to me and looking up to me about being qualified to compete at the upcoming 2013 CrossFit Games.

A. J. Roberts asked me if I had a sponsor yet, and I told him no. He said, "Why not? You are like a walking billboard for these folks." When I got home, I picked two sponsors I thought would be cool to sponsor me, and—lo and behold—they both said yes. I had sent them letters requesting a sponsorship and telling them what I had to offer. To this day, nearly four years later, I am still sponsored by 321 Apparel, Michael Shach. Through good and not-so-good times, this company has stood behind me with their love and amazing kindness and generosity. I am eternally grateful and can't say enough about 321. Their clothes are absolutely amazing; they are trendy and hold up to the most grueling workouts and washing. People always comment on how cute my workout clothing is. I faithfully wear that clothing for virtually every workout I do and for other purposes, too, such as teaching clinics. I picked up the Sox Box as a sponsor too for 2013. They are known for their cool knee-high socks. They made me personalized socks.

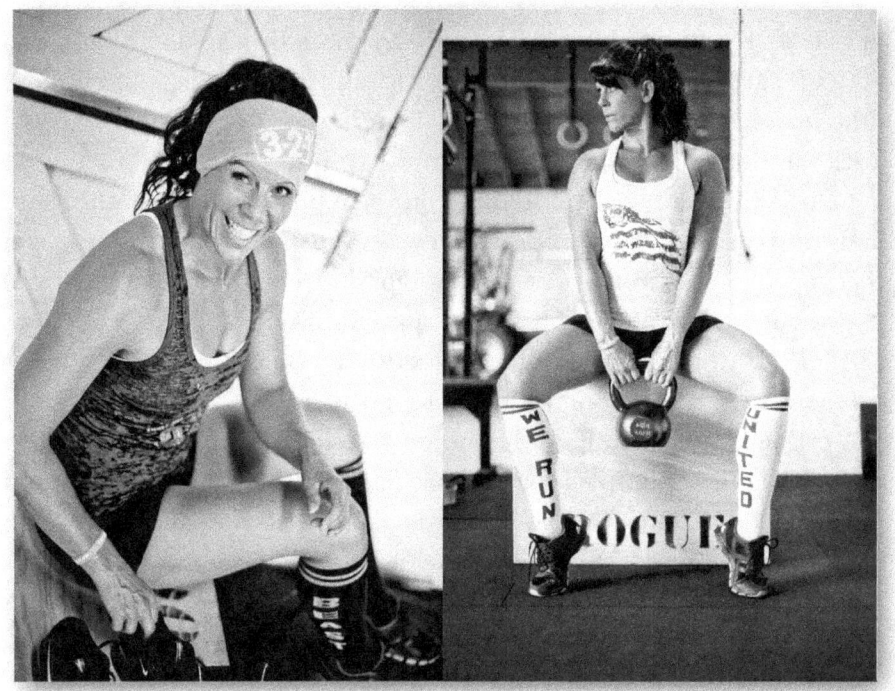

My sponsors 321 Apparel and Sox Box photo shoot 2013.

My sponsors required me to wear their clothing in different environments and turn in pictures and videos once a month so that they could use them in their social media. I wore their clothing during my workouts, as well as at the games in between events. In exchange for this, they paid for all my entry fees and supplied me with a ton of apparel. I never asked for more than that. I know other athletes who had their supplements and travel paid for, too. I was proud of my sponsors and what they did for me, and I loved their clothing so much that it was easy for me to wear it almost daily.

Training time flies between qualifying for the games and going to the games. My husband and I figured out that training for the games was going to require a lot more time to prepare. As ignorant as we were in that aspect, I knew I needed to dedicate more time to do my best, and we both agreed I needed to train as efficiently as possible to allow more time for recovery, work, and family. Training for one hour, five days a week was not making sense for the games training.

Earlier, we had decided to build our own box in a large building we had constructed on our property but weren't using. We were able to put that together in less than two weeks. For starters, Coach Jon was able to give me my private lessons out of that. Eventually, we expanded into further training. We called the box the Rodeo Blues Box because it was on the ranch called Rodeo Blues, where the barrel horses were raised and trained. So, basically, at that point, I would go into my original box and WOD with this special group Coach Rich had put together, and then I would take my OLY lessons twice a week at my box and work on a few special items. Then, as games got closer, I started double WODs per day. I would try to go to different boxes to WOD a second time with people and get different programing, as I had only one set of programming to rely on at that time. I was trying to prepare to be in better shape for games as I would WOD more than once a day—up to three times a day, actually. Training at different times was also a way to prepare for the different times of the day I would compete at during the games. Some of the other boxes around town also had different equipment, which provided me more variations. I was trying to prepare my body in as many ways as possible that I could think of. It was running mostly on common-sense ideas.

Competing at the games was insane to me. First, it was hard for me to believe I was even there. Most participants had been training far longer than I and had not come close to making it as a master or individual. My mother had told me I was getting a second chance to compete at a world level because having been sent home from the Olympic training center was a blessing. Funny, I had thought that myself several times, but her words solidified it. Here I was, and I barely knew what CrossFit entailed or what was about to happen. I knew God had put me into this situation because he had plans for me to share him to CrossFit people. My new field to evangelize in. I was excited about this.

It was hard not having any of my immediate family there other than my husband and daughter. What person competes at the world games and has little to no family support? Perhaps everything had happened so quickly, and my family knew what CrossFit was only because I suddenly was doing it. Going without their support gave me the opportunity to know what that felt like and taught me that I must always try to be there and support them so I know what their endeavors are. I would not have known this and how important it is had I not gone through it myself. I also knew that was all worldly support, and you cannot depend on that. I was reminded that I can depend on only God and myself.

Things started to sink in a little at the opening of the games when the event coordinators played "The Star-Spangled Banner." Emotions crept over me, and the tears streamed down my cheeks. I realized how blessed I was to be there and that I could share my lessons with people who wouldn't get this opportunity. I also became scared and finally thought, "This is about to go down right now. Have I done everything I should have done?"

I found out the answer to that sooner rather than later. One of my weaknesses was revealed during the handstand push-ups WOD. This is considered a gymnastics move because you are moving your own body weight in a handstand push-up against a Plexiglas wall. It actually combined two of my weaknesses at the time: body-weight movement and overhead strength. I came nowhere even close to finishing that WOD. I had done well before that, but those scores brought me down. Even with the two WODs I did well in, I still missed going to the finals by one point. Most people would think that just qualifying and going to the games was a huge accomplishment, especially in such a short time of CrossFitting, and that it was a place to go and have fun. I did not see it that way by any means. I needed to please certain people. And of course, I was highly disappointed in myself and my current training methods. This became the fuel for the training for 2014. I had to go back to the games and prove to myself and others that I could do much better. It became an obsession. From that moment on, I was living a CrossFit dream. My whole life revolved around CrossFit.

Generally speaking, I had a great experience at the games. I was pleased at the way headquarters ran everything. Our events were at the running track, which was a step up from parking lots in the past, I was told. They had a nice, big tent for the athletes that had air-conditioning and lots of space in which to rest and relax. Gravity chairs were available to pass out on. Personnel provided plenty of fresh water and healthy meals and snacks. The warm-up area was close and amply supplied with equipment to get a nice warm-up going. A medical area was available to us for first aid, mobility, massage, ice baths, and chiropractic care. Another section had food vendors and shopping vendors. The judges did an amazing job, along with all the other volunteers. It was easy to hear and figure out what was going on at all times. Programming for the events was well rounded. It fully tested me. I also liked the fact that it was free admission to watch the masters.

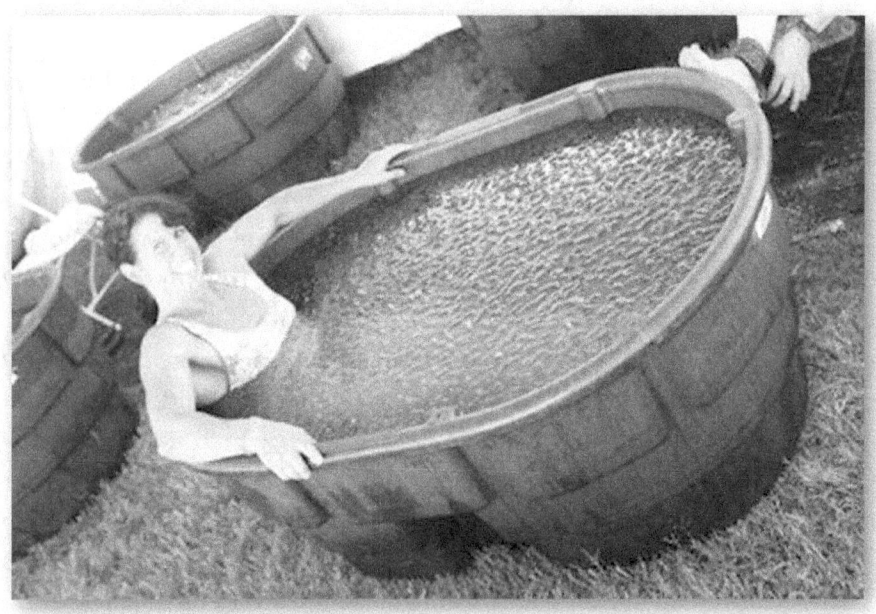

Ice bath at 2013 Games.

Another part of the games I hadn't planned on was the fact that you sort of become a superstar. Before competing, you have to go through a check-in process, and part of that process is receiving close to $4,000 to $5,000 worth of Reebok clothing. The organizers make it a personal, up close, and fun process. As you walk around in the hotel, heading toward the check-in process, people recognize you and say congratulations and that you're awesome. The hotel lobby is decorated for the games and Reebok. You start to feel special. Receiving all that colorful and trendy CrossFit gear from Reebok is overwhelming and joyful. I was surprised and grateful for the generous gifts. It lifted me and made me super excited to compete. It was a memory to not be forgotten or taken lightly. Reebok does require you to wear their gear while competing, but who wouldn't want to? Reebok has led the way for CrossFit clothing and gear, I am sure.

With Reebok being in contract with headquarters as their sponsor, they also control the photography. That was a bit of a problem because you want to bring a camera with a big-enough lens to take good close-ups, but they would not allow that, and they wouldn't offer their photos for sale. That was a bummer because you want the memories, and going to the games is definitely a time you want documented. I guess that would be one of my few complaints.

Even though I did not qualify to go to the finals, I placed thirteenth, and CrossFit took only twelve. I stayed and watched to learn. It certainly was a battle to the finish and quite fun to watch and strategize. It was another time to feel special because many people in the stands recognize you, come up and congratulate you, and say nice things. They also ask a lot of questions. "How long have you been doing CrossFit?" "Do you have a coach with you at the games?" "What was your training like?" And so on. I like to mention Coach Rich at the games. He was my first and main coach in getting me to the games. He was also willing to coach me there. He was like a completely different person there because he was so focused on me and my needs. I felt connected and was grateful for his sharpness in helping me get through all my events with confidence. It was a special time in my life I had with him, and no one can ever take that away. My husband, Randy, was also a huge support to me before, during, and even more so after the games. He also realized all the work that needed to be done to turn my weaknesses into strengths. He never left my side at the games except when he was forced to. People often ask me, "What was the coolest thing that happened to you at the games?" Well, the truth is that the games brought my husband and me closer together. I had never thought about our relationship growing deeper through CrossFit, but it did because the way he treated me showed me a side I never knew existed. He made everything so much easier for me and had my back on everything. I felt an incredible amount of love and dedication from this man that I hadn't expected. To me, that was my everything that I brought back from the games in 2013. To this day, I am still inclined to answer that question the same way.

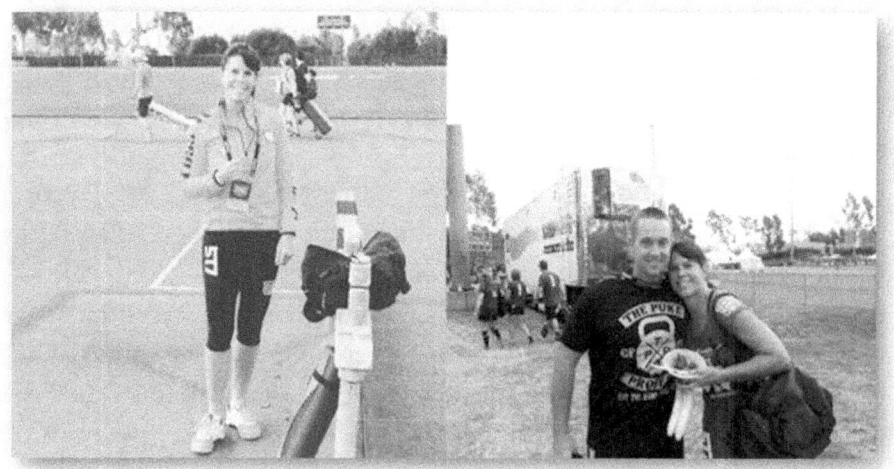

2013 CrossFit Games and Coach Rich.

Somehow, in the midst of all this training and competing, I managed to acquire a fan base. I am not sure if those people know how important they are in getting an athlete to the top like that. I do think that some of them know because many times, just at the right moments, they said or did the right things that pushed me through dark spots I had to get through to go forward. These people were angels showing up out of the blue. Some of the things that stand out include receiving an uplifting text, seeing someone show up right before one of my grueling practices to watch and cheer me on, or having people jump in and train with me. What about those who pack up their vehicle with all their kids and travel a full day to watch me compete? They spend their hard-earned money on fuel, hotels, and food and then want to go out and eat with me after I've finished competing, regardless of what place I earned. They make it a point to tell me how proud they are of me, and it's genuine. Then, when something goes down less than perfectly, they have my back in more ways than I thought would occur. Wow. That's a pretty darn supportive fan base.

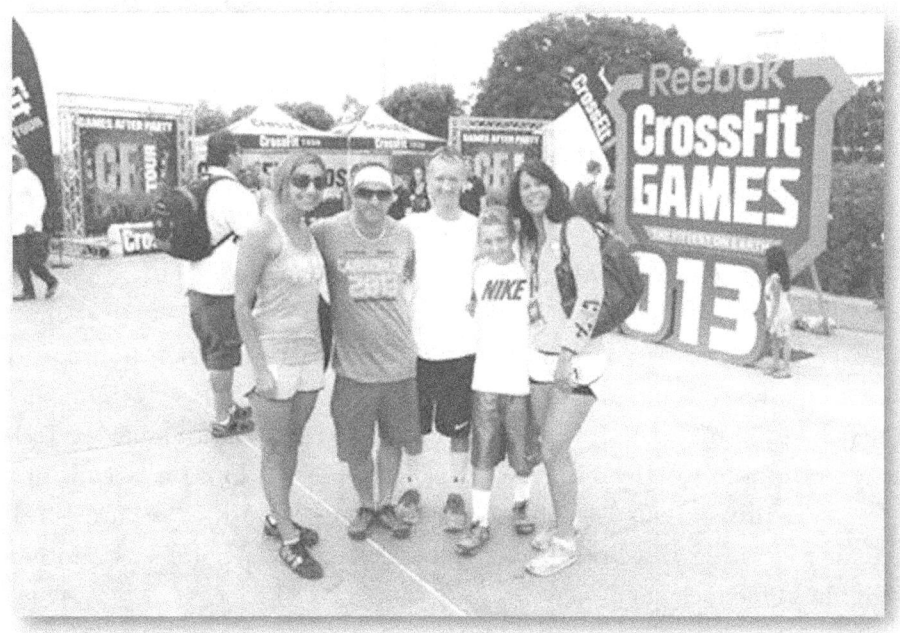

Some of my top fans that came to the games.

Those people have made my job easier. When they tell me that I inspire them, and they are only twenty-three years old, my heart surges with happiness because I love knowing that I am helping others become healthier both physically and mentally. Having a tiny bit of my family there and some close friends was also fulfilling inside my heart. They said they would not have missed me compete for the world and were so proud of me regardless of my finish. My daughter, Gabrieal, made me feel amazing by getting herself there with my grandson. They had to travel from one end of the state to the other to watch me live.

You don't think too much about it, but you are demonstrating for people how to make changes in their lives for the better while competing at the games. CrossFit is magical in that aspect; it's so amazing to watch people kick some physical butt, and then you go home and do it yourself because you are so pumped up. I believe it motivates others to go home and take their motivation to another level, even if they're not competitive. The energy at the games has a certain effect on people, just like the Olympics does. People want to better themselves after being fans at the games.

After competing at the games and staying to watch the master finish, we stayed on an extra day to watch the individuals compete, and we visited all the shopping areas. I also spent some time at 321 Apparel's booth with the owners, Michael and Phil. I was finally meeting them for the first time, as they are from Florida. I had a great time with them. I was completely dressed in their attire and hung around their booth, sort of modeling and meeting people coming in and out. It was there that they handed me one of my sponsor checks, which was an amazing feeling and photo worthy. Phil also stocked me up on more new clothing. I can't express enough as an athlete how important it is to have good-quality clothing to work out in. Meeting them in person was another highlight for me that week.

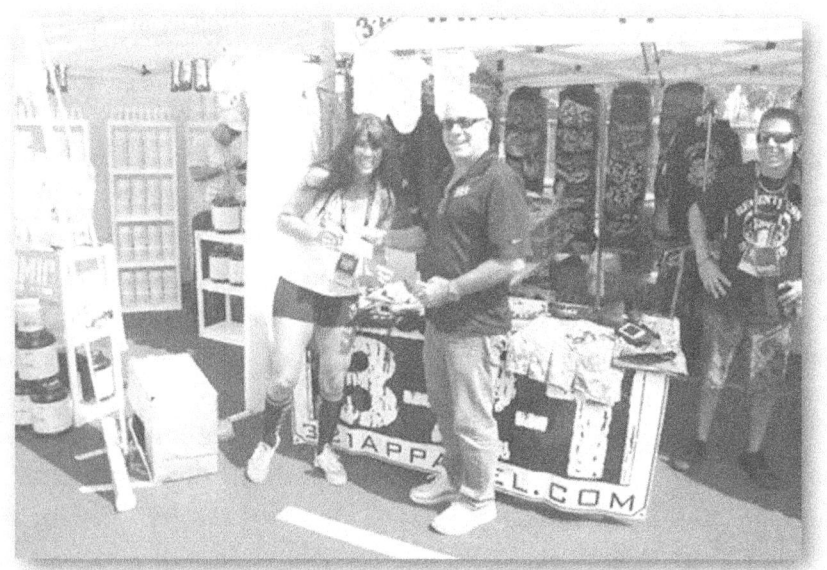

Spending time and receiving my sponsor check from 321 Apparel.

Being at the games so early on, my family and I were ready to start heading home to Redding. Years earlier, we had found a spot in Pismo Beach where we liked to vacation, so we decided to stop there on the way home and spend a few days on the beach, sipping champagne and checking out CrossFit boxes in the area. You would think I would want to take a break and rest, but I was still amped up. We tried CrossFit Grover Beach one day. After we were done working out, we talked for a few minutes with the owner, Ben Green. He said, "You guys should move here. I could be your coach. You can work out here for free, and I will pay you a dollar a month if you let me coach you."

It was too funny, but we were interested in moving to the ocean and closer to Southern California; we just didn't think we could afford to live near any body of water. Ben said his mom was a real estate agent and that we should call her. Later that day, I did just that, and she came to our hotel for a glass of coastal wine. We talked real estate. She said it was totally possible for us to be able to afford to live there. Randy and I could not believe this. Real estate was still pretty recessed, and prices were down; there was low inventory but enough to look at. We knew we would have to get the ranch sold in Redding, and that would be a real challenge because Redding was hit hard by the recession, and things were bouncing back very slowly. The cool thing is that Randy and I both knew that all things are possible in God. The hard part about that would be obeying his time frame. When we got back to Redding, we called our real estate friend and started the journey of preparing to put our house in Redding on the market.

Heading home from Pismo Beach to Northern California, I was already plotting and planning on how to approach the training for the open for 2014. I received a strong message that 2015 would be my year. Once I returned home, I shared this message with both of my coaches, and they both had the same response. They both said that while that may be the case, I had to try to make it back to 2014. I never said I wasn't going to try for 2014; rather, I was saying that 2015 would be my year. I knew that I had to put most of my training time into my weaknesses, which were gymnastics and overhead movements. I was planning to have a meeting with my OLY coach, Jon, on how to approach all this. My upper-body strength was weak, which is pretty common in women, but it can be overcome. I was thinking that rather than being strung out on three different boxes. I was going to have to make some changes and eliminate a box and a coach. This was going to be a painful experience for me because I was worried about hurting people's feelings. I was afraid that they would see me as being ungrateful for all the help they had given me and that they would ridicule me and judge me harshly. I can take things personally sometimes. Rather than considering what is in everyone's best interest, I have taken things way too personally and have reacted poorly and selfishly. I knew I was not alone in this type of behavior. After much thought, it was a no-brainer: I needed a full-time coach who was more experienced in teaching me the skills I needed help with and who was able and willing. I decided to train out of my box full time and have Jon further my coaching. He was coming twice a week, and we started adding more programing to my training sessions. I programmed around his programming and did more of what I thought I needed. I bought a punch card from his box and would pop in there several times a week and WOD with his peeps. It was insane how fast that training time went by.

Before competing in the games, I had seen a competition was coming up in the later part of August called the Oregon Summer Games 2013. I researched it and saw that they had a master forty-plus division. The dates seemed cool because I would have games experience at this point and still be in pretty good shape from the games training. It felt right to enter it. I shared the info with my coaches and other athletes, but no one was interested in it at all except me. It was only a five-hour drive from the house, and Bend, Oregon, is actually a nice place. I remember what Coach Rich had said about staying independent and not relying on him to be there, and he was right. I entered it on my own, knowing I would make the drive alone and sleep, eat, and compete alone. It turned out to be a good shot in the dark for me. I actually made my first podium appearance, which thrilled my sponsors. I met some cool people who shared and supported me in many ways, including Brian and Mary Oare. One of my best friends from Alaska was living in Oregon at the time, and he drove over and coached and supported me the first day I competed. This show was put on quite well. The prizes were great for making the podium, and the programing was true CrossFit style. There was awesome equipment to WOD on, good judges, and a great venue. I suggest the event add age groups every five years, like the games and NorCal Masters, to make it fair and competitive for the masters. I mean, I don't think a sixty-year-old master wants to compete against a forty-year-old master. I was fifty-three, and I competed against mostly forty-year-olds. I believe there was only one other female gamer, and she was slightly older than me. But I felt good because I had been unhappy with my finish at the games. I made the podium because I was consistent again.

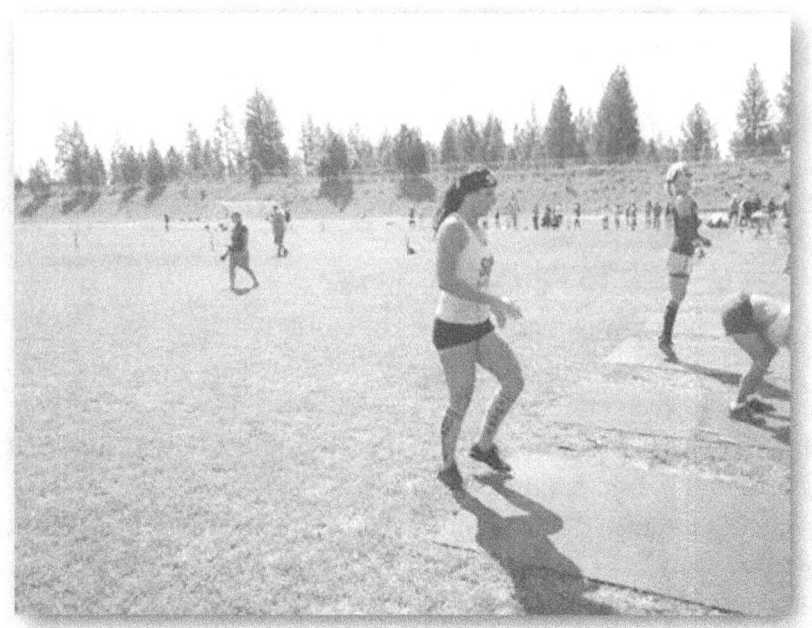

Competing at the Oregon Summer Games in 2013.

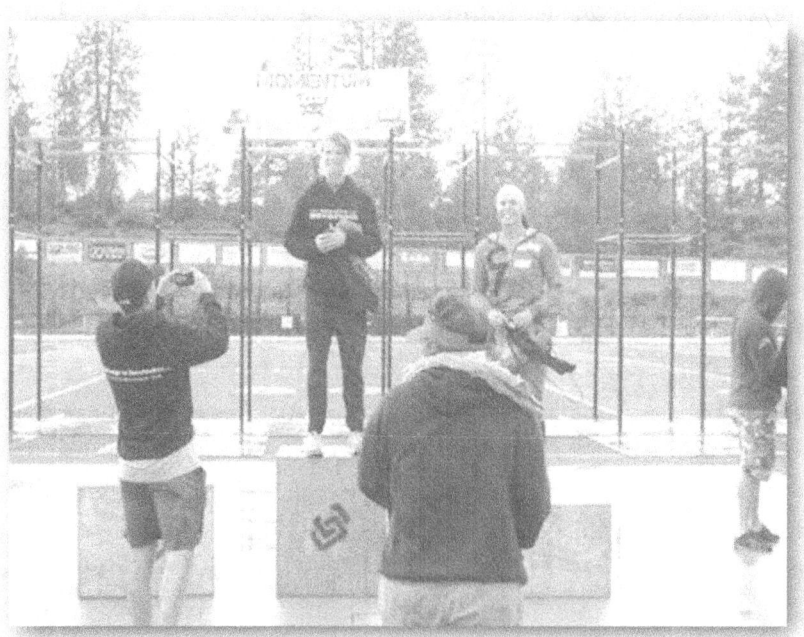

My first podium appearance, and in the rain!

CHAPTER 7

RECOVERY

FROM A NUTRITION standpoint, you can aid your recovery with both a pre-WOD drink and a post-WOD drink. Read your labels and research what you are putting into your body. It does not make any sense to put harmful ingredients into your body, especially since you're trying to optimize your health. You've got to ordain your diet completely around your training and recovery. Without a solid, optimized nutrition program, you won't have a maximally productive workout. To me, that means my diet has to be spot on, all the time. If I'm going to eat something off kilter, I need to plan it around my training program. My diet when I started CrossFit was strict Paleo: protein with every meal, lots of veggies, two pieces of fruit per day (I'm a big apple fan), and some nuts or seeds. I thought I was doing a good job. Coach Jon had tried to speak to me a few times about my diet. I thought I was good and wasn't open to his suggestions. A lot of that kind of attitude blockage comes from an issue I deal with about body weight and how I see myself. I also had some issues with bulimia in the past but had it under control. It wasn't in my best interest not to chat with him about it or go to a clinic, as he suggested. Thankfully, I had someone else looking out for me, too.

After you drink your recovery shake, it's important you hit your process of mobility. Working on your ROM for your joints can be boring, time consuming, and painful. Doing mobility on a regular basis is a top priority in more than just the obvious recovery phase. If your ROM is limited, you will max out on, say, a snatch weight and stay there because your limited ROM will prevent you from getting into the correct position. Many people get injured outside the box because they are not addressing their mobility needs. Some people may be so tight that they jump out of their truck and—whoops!—they tear their groin. Perhaps on that day they did a lot of sumo dead-lift high pulls and didn't take the time to take care themselves, and jumping out of the truck caused an over usage injury.

When I started addressing mobility with myself, I didn't find too many coaches in CrossFit who knew much about or even addressed it. I knew it was important, and Coach Jon had brought it up to me several times. I also realized again that I was responsible for my own mobility, and it had to be addressed. I decided to get my mobility CrossFit certification so that I could learn more about it, meet more amazing people, become certified to teach it, and have my issues discovered. I began the work.

Deciding where to go to take the certification was easy. I wanted to take it with the guru Dr. Kelly Starrett at his box in San Francisco. He's a physical therapist who has taken physical therapy to the highest level possible, from preventative to recovery. He teaches the mobility courses for CrossFit headquarters and has his own box in San Francisco. He has written several books (*Becoming a Supple Leopard*, *Ready to Run*, and *Deskbound*) and has developed many mobility tools. These are just a few of his accomplishments, I'm sure.

Going to his certification course turned out to be a real trip. I made the mistake of letting him know I had gone to the games in 2013, and suddenly I became his example in front of a large group of people. I'm pretty sure he found a lack of ROM in every joint in my body over the next two days for everyone else to see. As embarrassing as it was, it was great to know all my issues up front, close and personal, so I could start addressing them as quickly as possible. However, being used as an example took away from some of my learning experience. Many times, I was on the floor, facedown or turned around, and he was demonstrating on me, which put me in a position where I could not see what was going on or what the fix was.

I combatted that when I returned to Redding by taking personal mobility lessons with Kevin Vance Suttmoeller for seven to eight weeks in my own private box. It was easy for him to identify my lack of ROM in just about every joint. He showed me a variety of exercises, superpartners (people who help you get in a position you cannot do alone), stretches, and roll outs and applied pressure with lacrosse balls for myofascial release. After we got my prescription down, my hourly routine with him was a brief warm-up to get the blood flowing (e.g., a four-hundred-meter row). Then, starting with the toes, we worked our way up to the top of the body, all in one hour. If you take mobility seriously, what needs to be done will differ from person to person. You adapt your mobility with your workouts, your schedule, and what you need for recovery. I think mobility is a nice piece to an active-rest day.

An active-rest day is another aid in recovery. Getting out and doing something, like going for a short hike or swimming a few laps to help you stay loose and remove toxins while still resting, is very helpful. I think that staying out of the box on your rest day is wise, for you can get burned out. But if weather inhibits you, you can do some mobility indoors for active rest. Just remember that you're resting, so don't take your mobility to a workout mode. Get in, get it done, and get out. Let your brain think about something else besides CrossFit, too.

Another pointer in improving your recovery involves supplementation. You can take supplements to help aid the body in reducing inflammation, allowing you to recover quicker. Many kinds of supplements exist, but one that is in the forefront is fish oil. Omega-3 fatty acids can help with joint swelling and reduce inflammation. COQ10 is another vitamin that can reduce swelling, along with bromelain, which is from pineapple. The choices are plentiful, and many of these supplements have multiple positive effects on the body. It is our responsibility to find out what we need and what works best for us. The supplement list is endless.

Massage is also a huge aid in recovery. When preparing for the games, I have had up to two deep tissue massages per week. They are not cheap, but boy do they pay off. Increasing the circulation in your body rids the toxins quicker, allowing the soreness to subdue faster. A good deep-tissue masseuse can work out knots that could be preventing your full potential or causing pain. He or she can be a superpartner and help stretch you into positions you can't get into yourself, thereby increasing your ROM. If you are able to relax and allow the process to happen, you get stress relief. Getting massages on a regular basis may be a huge key in reducing or preventing injury. Once you find a good masseuse and you see him or her on a regular basis, you can often get a reduced rate. For me, the massages were a huge reward from working hard, and they were huge in my recovery and reaching my full potential as an athlete. I could not have gone to the games without this piece of recovery.

Chiropractic care is also crucial in recovery and in helping stay injury free. Correcting spinal alignment and function can maximize our performance and help reduce injuries. As athletes, we deal with asymmetry—one side of the body being stronger than the other or mobility and flexibility issues. The chiro can help us align through adjustments. If we can stay balanced or aligned, it will keep us from overusing one side or part of the body and then breaking down into injury. Misalignments slow down the body from recovery. Chiro adjustments allow the body to move freely, as it was designed to. I have had great relief from chiropractic care all my life. My grandmother was a great proponent of it, and she passed that on to me.

Soaking in tubs with essential oils and Epsom salt is helpful in so many ways. Essential oils are absorbed right into our skin (our largest organ) and can also be absorbed through diffusors. You can take some orally, just make sure they are food grade. It's worth taking a look at essential oils and their healing effects. You can find them for every situation, from reducing inflammation to sleeping better. I highly recommend them. Some of the companies make a great muscle rub, which is amazing stuff. You can get super savvy with these oils and make your own muscle rubs.

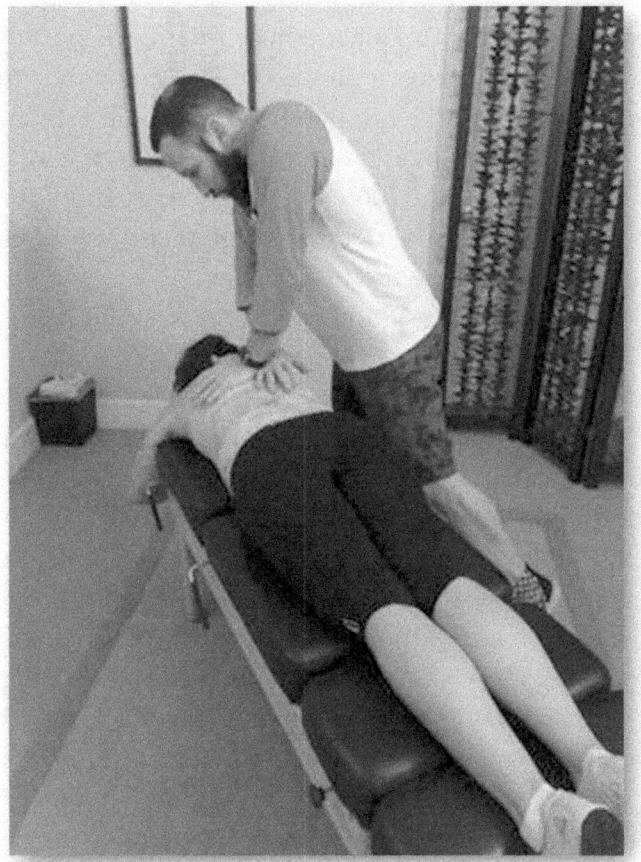

Dr. B. adjusting me weekly.

Yoga and Pilates are huge in removing toxic waste and alleviating soreness as part of the recovery process. They also put you into a peaceful mental state and remove you from the worries of the world for an hour. Another benefit is that they help increase your flexibility or your ROM. Some of the more advanced Pilates studios that do one-on-one or small-group sessions actually have apparatuses that assist the athlete. Two of the many pieces of equipment are called reformers and cadillacs. These aid by removing body weight, which helps you get into positions you could not get into otherwise. They can also add resistance. I found these machines to be extremely helpful in stretching and increasing strength in minute amounts. That can make a huge difference in your lifts, all by increasing your ROM. Pilates is also about learning to breathe through the entire movement, working on both inhaling and exhaling by using all your abdominal muscles and other muscles in your core area. Using the correct Pilates breathing route, you engage core strength and utilize your lungs way more. You also detox through them. More oxygen equals more energy.

Rest is maybe the biggest and most necessary aid in recovery. You have got to sleep and rest. Get off your feet, and kick back. Get your butt in bed early enough to ensure you get all the sleep that your body needs to recover. Put your phone in a different room, and for goodness sake, turn it off. A caller will leave a message if it is important, and Facebook, Twitter, and Instagram won't miss you, I promise. You have to figure out for yourself what it takes to get proper rest. I am not a napper, but that may be how you can get some of your rest. I go to bed early and sleep for hours and hours on end without any aid of any sort. If you have a good exercise routine going or a competitive-athlete routine going, you need eight to twelve hours of rest. Coach Jon said a good night's rest is when you sleep well and don't wake up until you wake up naturally—not with an alarm. I think this is the ideal situation for rest. I know it's not easy to get that much sleep, but if you want to be healthy, you have to make rest a priority.

CHAPTER 8

COMPETITIVE TRAINING

As I HAD mentioned earlier, after the 2013 games, we started increasing the training volume. I could not get through it without the recovery modules. For the most part, I was pretty diligent about it, especially the mobility parts. It worked best to address a little bit of it when I would first start my work out daily and then all of it that needed to be done when I was finished. What I would target when I first started to train was based on my lifts that day and how sore I was. Training at this level could be lonely, and I know there are high-level athletes reading this right now who totally know what I mean. I was always the last to leave. Coach Jon had graciously opened up a high-caliber athlete-training time at the box without instruction but still under his amazing programing. At the time, he was using a lot of the Outlaw Way style of programming. There would be five or six of us on some days but only a few on most other days. At the time, I did not realize how priceless this was to have these athletes to train with. If you can get anybody to train with you for two to three hours per day, day in and day out, you are double blessed. Not many people can put that kind of time in or even want to address that much time in the box. I do get that.

I was elated when Jon invited me to join this group because I knew this was the cream of the crop in Redding. Little did I know, I was about to step into the arena of the hardest training I had ever done in my life, which was soon to be a way of life and a full-time job. The group varied in age and gender, but I was by far the oldest. Yet I was definitely fit and talented enough to hang strongly with them, rarely finishing last in the metcons (metabolic conditioning). The training sessions were usually about two to two and a half hours long. With the added mobility, I was in that session for a good, solid three hours per day. This type of hardcore training turned my sleeping pattern from seven to eight hours per night to ten to twelve, hitting thirteen on an occasion or two. The full-time job consisted of training, journaling the training, preparing meals and snacks, grocery shopping, eating, resting, using recovery methods including mobility, studying programing, and sleeping. I had little time for anything else, and the rest days were filled with catching up on everything that needed to get done: housework, yard work, working, etc. I needed to be highly organized to keep up, and I was.

The programming was at times unbelievable. On some days, I would look at it and cringe. We would all encourage one another and get through it. I was strong enough by then that I could about RX it all, even as an aged master. *RX* is the prescription for the programming without scaling back, which is designed for individuals thirty-nine and younger. Training with the heavier RX weights was painful. The result was when the weights were dropped back to meet my age bracket requirements during competition, it was easier. Wall ball weights for me were twenty pound balls and ten foot targets. Very difficult movement that made the twelve pound ball and nine foot target feel like a toy game at the competition. We all took turns crawling out of the gym, except Coach Jon. The poor guy had to stay and teach several classes after that. The crew that met at this time started out with a good number of competitive athletes; unfortunately, the numbers dwindled fast. Committing that amount of time is time consuming in itself, but what it does to the body is a whole other story. As I mentioned early, it's a full-time job. Many days saw only a handful of us. People have to be able to function in their work and take care of their families. It got lonely very quickly. This is where having discipline and being a self-starter are excellent qualities to be born with, because no one showed up on some days. It didn't matter how many were there; I was going to work out and finish it, with others or alone, at the very best I could do. I realized how blessed I was to be in a position where I could make this a priority in my life. So many others wanted to but were not in the same position. This is yet another affirmation that I am where God wants me to be, as he blessed me with the possibility to be in all of it.

When you train this hard with such regularity, the PRs keep coming. The saying "practice makes perfect" was definitely paying off in my book. Things were changing rapidly, including my body. When I initially started CrossFit, I weighed about 138 to 140 pounds. I was eating enough to maintain my weight. I am just over five foot seven. I prefer a smaller frame on myself, but that wasn't going to work out training the way I was to become stronger.

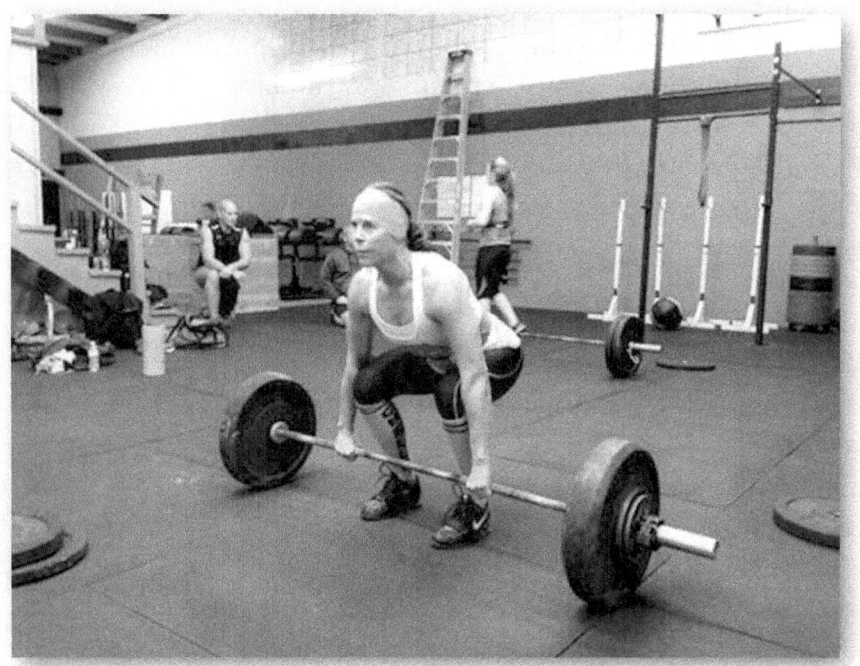

Training heavy and bulking up in preparation for the 2014 CrossFit Open.

Coach Jon recognized this first and told me to start eating a lot more. Eating enough to get by and eating clean was not going to be enough to get me to the games and keep me getting stronger. He told me to eat! I kept my diet clean but went from eating three meals per day with two snacks to six meals per day and snacks as needed. The muscle packed on, along with a little fat. The strength kept coming. The way I felt when working out when I increased my calories was great. I had so much more energy, and recovery was better because I wasn't dragging so much. I managed to put on about fifteen pounds rather quickly, and I put on more as time went by. It affected my training in only a positive manner. But mentally, I didn't feel good. I've been self-conscious about my figure my whole life. Becoming larger was difficult regarding clothing, too. Pants would fit nicely at the waist, but I could not get them over my thighs or hips. I found it easier not to step on the scale anymore.

This is common in CrossFit for women. My husband loved it. Being from the South, he prefers the bulk over the bones any day. My food types were mainly meat, seafood, fish, protein powders (both whey and vegan), vegetables, fruit, nuts, seeds, and oatmeal. I usually would do the oatmeal in the morning with protein powder, nuts, coconut milk, powdered greens, and cinnamon. Increasing my calories in a clean method was a huge part of my success in reaching my goals. Mentally, I was able to get over the size and settle into the benefits. I have to say, if a woman asked me if lifting or CrossFit makes her bulky, my answer would be that it depends on her diet and what level of CrossFit she commits to. You can do CrossFit and tone nicely and build some strength, but if you want to compete in CrossFit and do really well, you are going to have to eat—and yes, you will become bulky. Bulky with muscles is not so bad. Bulky is the new sexy, right? The other thing that happens that is typical while eating for strength and recovery is that my metcons got harder. As you are growing and getting bulkier, it is harder to mover quicker, unless it's a heavy barbell move. To keep up with my old metcon times, I had to find another gear that I didn't know I still had in me. It was uncomfortable, to say the least. I was out of that comfort zone and recovering flat on my back, making sweat angels! One of my fortes is metcons—the longer, the better. I can just go, big engine forever. It was difficult to keep the speed intact with size, though, on those metcons. I was finding my way by giving and taking.

I was also fortunate enough to have my husband to train with in our private box at home. He was just starting to get into CrossFit at this point. There was a time he rebuked it. The ten years he did in the military burned him out in the exercise field, but he was starting to come around as he watched my body and mind morph into something neither of us thought would be possible for a fifty-three-year-old. I felt as if he wanted a piece of that; plus, I know he wanted to spend that time with me. His job required him to be away from home two weeks of each month, so when he was home, we needed to make the most of it. He was already eating a Paleo diet while at home, and the weight was dropping off him. When he started CrossFit, it came off even quicker, and the muscle started to pack on. He lost sixty pounds and then put on about twenty pounds of muscle. He is down forty pounds and has gone from a 38 waist to a 32 to 34—amazing! I'm so proud of this guy. When we started training together, it was a little tough on me because I am not the most patient person with family. Sometimes, I would get frustrated with him when I had to show him something for the third time. It wasn't uncommon for Coach Jon to show me something twelve times, but that was different. The thing that really impressed me is my husband's perseverance and motor. He does not quit, and he can focus. He would sometimes complain to me about the programming, and I would explain why we had to do it. When he would continue to complain (because he believed something was wrong with it, whether it was my programming or Coach Jon's), I finally said, "Look, no one is holding a gun to your head and making you do this." He stopped whining after hearing that a few times. Besides Coach Jon, he is the best training partner ever. He's dedicated and committed.

When we built our own private box, many people showed interest in it and asked if they could come and WOD with us. We always said yes. When they would show up, we would tell them we were on a hard training program, and by no means did we expect them to do what we were doing. They could scale down or do their own thing, and we were just happy to have them at Rodeo Blues Box. Not one of them ever did anything else but what our program was, and very few of them ever returned. The training was no joke and just plain not attractive for your average athlete. Again, it's a lonely road out there at that training level. Never in my athletic career have I ever trained that hard, or so I thought. This is about the time my body started sleeping ten to twelve hours per night.

When the 2014 open rolled around, my entire team (as far as I knew) thought I was prepared once again to make it to the games. I had put my whole life on hold, from giving up riding horses professionally to spending way less time with my family, missing out on many family-and-friend functions. I struggled through the open and discovered I was not even close to being ready. I did not make it back to the games.

CrossFit headquarters was getting a lot of complaints from the master divisions, which are from age thirty-nine and above. People thought CrossFit should be giving the masters more opportunity to compete than just at the high level of the games. For example, the individuals from ages eighteen to thirty-nine have an extra competition called regionals, which qualifies them for the games. Those are executed in different regions of the world, and this gives more people the opportunity to compete at a professional event outside of the games. The masters were wanting a piece of that, so CrossFit changed the qualifying status of the masters to get to the games. Instead of being the top twenty in an age bracket, they went to being in the top two hundred and then participating in the masters' qualifying round. Those top twenty would go to the games.

I placed twenty-first in the open and forty-third in the masters' qualifying round. I scored so low in the latter because Crossfit headquarters programed muscle-ups (MUPs), and I did not have MUPs, along with many other master women in my age group. That is a men's gymnastics move on a set of rings, requiring pull and a push mostly from upper-body strength. One of my weaknesses is body-weight movement. You can do them either strict or "kipping." (A kip is a transference of movement first generated in the horizontal plane to the vertical plane, where momentum and a perfectly timed pull from the back launch the athlete forcefully upward.) I could not do either, and little or no practice was available because I was so new to CrossFit and did not have a gymnastics background. The danger of injury was high. I was not strong enough at that point. So, I had to sit the games out.

I think when I came back from the 2013 games, I realized maybe once or twice I was one of the oldest girls—if not the oldest in my age bracket—who made it to the games that year. I didn't think anything about it before the games because I was so ignorant about CrossFit that I had no clue it mattered. It was perhaps a good thing mentally. After looking at the stats of the top twenty of the master qualifiers for 2014, I saw it was mainly the youngest in that age group who qualified. It made me realize that having my next birthday and turning fifty-five was going to allow me to be one of the babies of the late-fifties age group. This was another affirmation that 2015 was going to be my year.

Well, I think everyone was shocked that I did not make it to the games in 2014. It was a sad day. Many of us at the box were on pins and needles waiting for the scores to come in and hoping they wouldn't move me down. Then, it happened: I was moved out of the top-twenty position. I remember walking around the corner of the box my coach owned, and we about ran into each other. The first thing that came out of his mouth was, "I am sorry!" I think at that moment we both felt a little failure in us. I didn't cry until I saw him. We hugged, and I made that long drive home.

The drive was interesting. I felt a sense of relief in many ways, which was surprising. I guess I didn't realize how much pressure I had put on myself until that moment when it suddenly lifted, and I felt free. I thought I could finally take a break and not feel guilty because I had earned the time off. But in the back of my mind, I was already figuring out the new plan. Part of the plan was to head to the games and watch my competition. I had asked Coach Jon about the new plan. Even though I requested to him that I return to the box the following week to start the new plan, he told me most people go home and rest for two weeks or so. That's what I had to do.

I wanted to study my competitors in the next age group and learn more about the games, looking in from outside the competition. That's why I decided part of my new training plan was going to the games as a spectator. I guess another reason why I may have been relieved was because I also knew I wasn't supposed to go back until 2015, and now I didn't have to try so hard to do something that wasn't in God's plan for me. Of course, none of it was done in vain. I was already preparing for 2015 as I had prepared for qualifications in 2014 and was becoming a very well-rounded CrossFit master athlete. I also believed I did not let anybody down because my team, sponsors, family, and friends knew how hard I had trained during that year after the 2013 games. I had also managed to stay injury free. That was huge. I mean, I had minor bumps and strains, but nothing took me out of my game at this point. I had about two years of solid CrossFit by then.

While we were at the games in 2014 as spectators, something amazing happened. We had just arrived at the StubHub Center and were getting settled in. I was looking over the program and was drawn to a one-hour gymnastics clinic that CrossFit headquarters was putting on for free in the staging area. The almighty Jeff Tucker was teaching it. I had not taken the gymnastics certification in CrossFit yet and had just signed up for it in Anchorage, Alaska—my hometown—and put half a deposit down. These certifications are no joke, and they are not cheap. As I was reading about the seminar, I reminded myself that I was not very good in gymnastics, and there would be a ton of young people there who were far more flexible and body-weight stronger than me. I was talking myself out of going to watch or enroll in this free, hour-long clinic. I was convincing myself that the staging area where they would have it would be brutally hot and uncomfortable. I actually looked at the brochure three times, trying to talk myself out of it each time. It was to start in ten minutes. After the third time of looking at the brochure, I shared it with my husband. He stood up, grabbed my hand, and said, "Let's go!" I was shocked and had no time to talk him out of it. We ran over to the area and quickly signed up and started the clinic with about fifty people. Yes, we were by far the oldest and the least gymnastics fit. We both made it through the clinic. In the end, Jeff Tucker, the CrossFit headquarters head gymnastics instructor, announced to the entire class that we would all receive a *free* CrossFit course certification anywhere we wanted to go. If we already had our certification, we could give it away to someone else. What? Unbelievable. What a blessing. I was already signed up for the course, and CrossFit headquarters refunded me my deposit. So, I was signed up for the course in Anchorage in September of 2015 for free! God never ceases to amaze me. It was a reward for being vulnerable and putting myself out on the line in front of lots of people who were adequate in gymnastics.

It was interesting watching the master women compete. It always appears different when you're looking from the outside in. Some looked to be breezing through at ease, and others looked to be suffering hard. I mainly focused on my age group, studying each one of those women. I also cheered on two of the competitors from my hometown. Both of my past and present coaches had one of their parents in the masters, and they were both good friends of mine. They both did very well, and I was proud of them. In some ways, I was relieved to be sitting this one out and observing and learning. You can feel the pain as a previous competitor watching them compete, and it made me nervous for them and myself. Then, I wished it was me out there, and I was excited to get home and restart the training to get back to the world CrossFit Games 2015. That was a goal I would be relentless about.

CHAPTER 9

OVERTRAINING

OVERTRAINING CAN BE tricky. Everyone responds differently when training intensely. When we set our minds to accomplish something, we don't always recognize things are happening around and in us because we are so focused on the prize. That's where a good coach can keep you out of trouble by always checking in with you to see how things are going, both mentally and physically. The programming he or she prescribes to you is crucial. Experience pays off, too, because you can recognize if you have gotten into some overtraining. As I mentioned before, everyone is different, but some of the signs of overtraining are not being able to sleep, loss of appetite, injuries (both minor and major), depression, constant soreness, poor attitude (especially before starting your training session), declining performance, feeling worn out or tired all the time, and more.

It's important that we do everything we can to avoid this while still riding the line to get the most out of our training. It takes time to figure this all out. Listening to your coach and your own body, while also being honest and backing off when necessary, can save you from a possible injury or mental burnout. Making sure you are recovering to recover (implementing recovery tools) can provide a lot of answers, provide preventative measures, and keep you on your A game for longer to grab that prize. When you have a hard work ethic like I do, even taking a rest day can be a mental challenge. When your coach tells you to go home and get some rest on a training day, do it. Your coach knows what is going on, and more than likely he or she has been there or has experienced it with another athlete. Find a way to relax your mind, and get it away from the gym every day. Take short trips that can give you a break from the monotony of training but still put you in a position where you can be physically active. You could even train in an out-of-town CrossFit box.

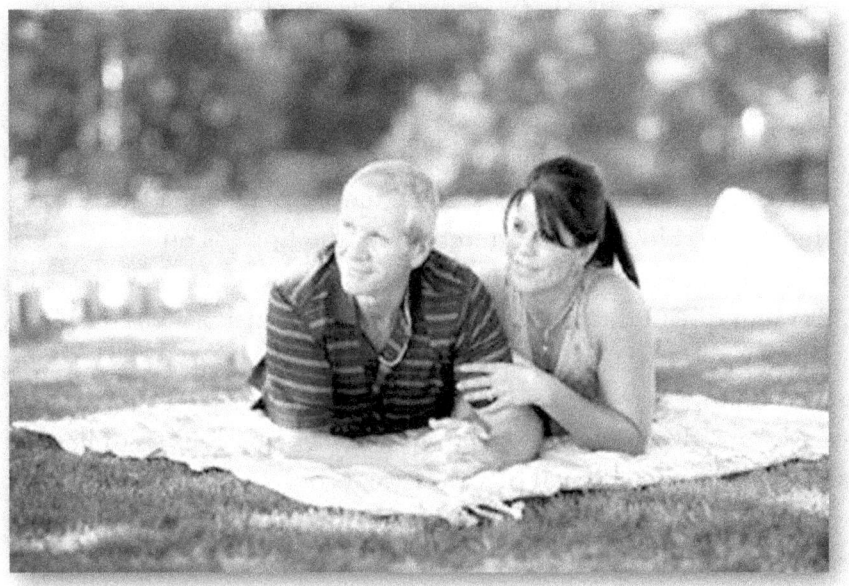

Relaxing in Lake Tahoe with my husband, Randy.

I found that in Pismo Beach. We had put the house up for sale in Redding, and we were patiently waiting for God to open the door and provide a buyer. We would take little trips to Pismo to look at houses for sale and also train in the CrossFit Grover Beach box, as there was a strong possibility that Ben Green would be my games coach for 2015. I had also signed up for my gymnastics certification in a different state, so that would mix up the training atmosphere a little bit.

CHAPTER 10

GOD IN ACTION

ALLOWING, WATCHING, AND knowing as God steers you in your current life affairs is amazing. Being able to share his unfoldment for you to others makes my heart thump. He has removed me from a field of barrel racing, where I joyfully ministered about the Lord as often as I was led, and placed me into a field of hardcore CrossFitters at a world-class level. This was a sport I did not know existed. I never had a clue that this was coming until I had received a message while barrel racing in Arizona to enter a bikini barrel race. About two weeks after getting that message, I received an advertisement to apply to enter a contest. I knew I had to fill out the paperwork, even at fifty-three years old. It was a road I was being led down. God is unbelievable at times, guiding us the entire time and helping us fulfill our dreams. Did I say amazing? Hearing him speak to me and obeying him can be challenging. The payoffs are rewarding, though.

My husband and I had taken the house off the market in January of 2015 and were planning to relist it in the spring, as suggested by our real estate agent. We thought that was a good idea because we were not getting many showings. My husband and I both knew in our hearts that the house would sell in God's timing, but I think we were both still trying to control it. We were having garage sales, cleaning stuff up, and getting stuff to the Salvation Army in case it sold. We did relist in the spring, and at that point I finally came to a place in my heart where I had given the sale of the house to the Lord. Instead of telling people I had done that, I was actually living it, and apparently so had Randy. In September, we were headed to Alaska for my CrossFit certification course in gymnastics, which I had won at the games and teach a competitive clinic. Before leaving for Alaska, we were working out in our private box. We were finishing up a two-hour session that Coach Jon had programmed for me when my friend Lois pulled up in her truck unannounced with a ton of moving boxes. I was kind of put out because I was hot, tired, and hungry, and I knew my husband would immediately want to put those boxes up in the box's loft because the house had not sold yet, and we were not packing. He would not want them sitting around for any period; it's the way he rolls. I thanked my good friend Lois for the boxes. Talk about surrounding yourself with positive and motivated people—well, Lois is one of them. She helped me and held my hand in so many ways. We put up all the boxes up in the loft as a team—hot, sweaty, tired, and hungry. I wondered why those boxes had suddenly arrived.

I had planned to stay two weeks in Alaska because that would allow me to fly in and out with my husband. He was working in the oil fields of Alaska on a two-week-on/two-week-off schedule. I also planned to spend time with family and friends while I was there. In addition, I put on a clinic on competitive training at CrossFit Anchorage, which received a great turnout. In exchange for training at CrossFit Anchorage, I coached a few of the classes and ran the open gym. That box treated me well and gave me free rein. I cannot express how much this meant to me. Vic and his box were a big part of my success. Vic was so warm and friendly and very respectful to me, along with his wife, Katy. They both had recently moved to Anchorage and opened their first CrossFit box.

The gymnastics clinic was awesome. That was my fifth certification, and haven't regretted any of them. I walked away from all of them with a ton of improvement in so many ways. I appreciate being able to learn to teach movements that maybe I can't do myself for one reason or another. However, I learned how to teach the movements, step by step, to others. I like learning about the scaled portion of the movement and accessory work to complement strength to acquire the movement.

Getting these certifications was important to me because you can learn so much about yourself and the others surrounding you. Who knew there was so much information to teach in a gymnastics-certification clinic in two days? I am sure that was the condensed version. Learning is a never-ending process.

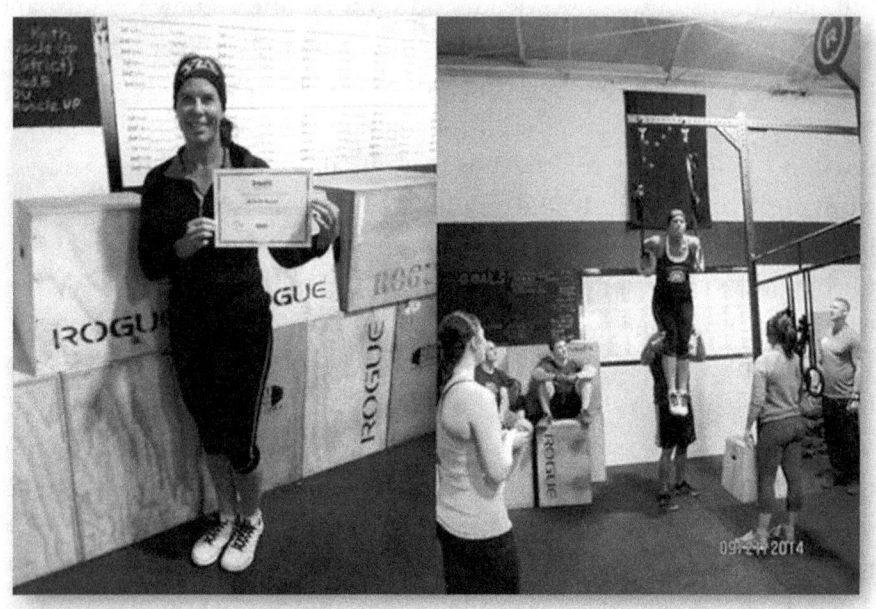

CrossFit gymnastics certification seminar held
at CrossFit Anchorage Alaska 2014.

About half my time had passed in Alaska. I got through the gymnastics clinic and was training hard every day with Coach Jon's personal programming for me. I even made some PRs while there and coached a lot. Then, I got a call from California. It was our real estate agent. She had a cash offer on our house in Redding with a thirty-day escrow. It suddenly dawned on me why the boxes showed up with Lois! My husband and I returned home after two wonderful weeks in Alaska and scrambled to make the move to the beautiful central coast of California, closer to the games and with a better climate to train in. Everything fell right into place. We knew God was working in our lives. All doors were open.

CHAPTER 11

TRAINING THROUGH ADVERSITY AND CHANGE

I TRAINED RIGHT up to the day we left Redding and started retraining shortly after we arrived in Pismo Beach. I took Ben Green up on his offer to make CrossFit Grover Beach my new affiliate box and have him as my third CrossFit coach. His mom was able to find us a lovely home at a reasonable price, and we were able to close on it and move in fairly quickly. I had a meeting with Ben because we both needed to know what we expected out of one another. We all agreed that Coach Jon needed to continue programming for me up through the games because he knew all my weaknesses and strengths. I told Ben I was very motivated but that he was not required to be with me at practice. I would appreciate any help he could give me, though, especially on technique, when he was around. We have a great relationship. Ben is easygoing and a loving, gifted, and talented athlete. I had been to his small, quaint box many times after the 2013 games, and I always felt right at home. I came from large boxes, so this was different for me. I easily got to know everyone rapidly, and I felt a strong sense of freedom and less pressure. Having less pressure did not take away my drive for training hard; it actually relaxed me and aided me in focusing and performing better.

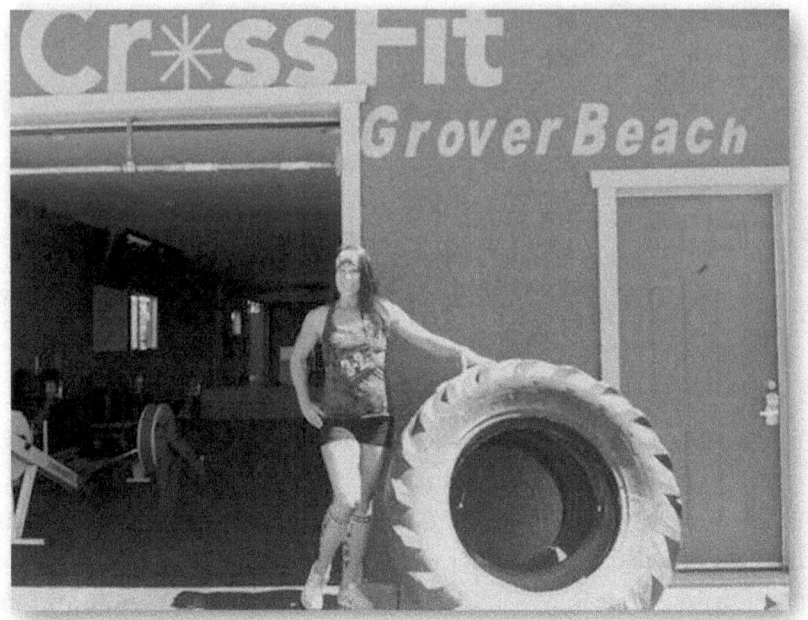

My 2015 affiliate CrossFit Grover Beach Box owned by Coach Ben Green.

I made sure I did not let the move or transition from Redding to Pismo Beach interrupt my training cycles. I made training my number-one priority and stayed organized to get everything done. That was well executed, and we were back into the full-time training mode with little downtime. The open was fast approaching, and the training was crucial and grueling. Ben was accommodating and made sure I had everything I needed and that things were in working order. When he had the time, he would stay over after his classes and look in on my training, giving tips where needed. I was able to oblige him by coaching his classes when he needed me. Sometimes, I would come in early and help his mom clean the box. Most of my training was done after normal class hours, so I did not interfere with his CrossFit classes. This was for the best, and I liked it, but boy it could be lonely. Randy was capable of training with me only when he was in town during his two weeks off. With the commute, he was training with me about ten days of the month. The programming was taking me about two and a half hours to get through and then another thirty minutes of mobility. I would have been so happy for any member who would come in and train with me because it was so much nicer to have someone there with me. Several people did just that.

I can recall when the class before my training time was over and everyone would clear out. It was as if a dark cloud would cover me, and I had to ignore it and work through it. It is not about work ethic or drive. I have only one gear: not stopping until I am done. It was simply a lonely, depressed, dark feeling. Having gone through this, I always want to offer to train with anyone who is going through anything similar. I know it's not something exclusive to me because Coach Jon and I have talked about this plenty. He has also been through the times of training alone.

As the training became grittier, it was pertinent I locate a good chiropractor in the new area I had moved to. I was already starting to feel misaligned, and lower-back pain was becoming my best friend. It was not from dead lifts. I felt God leading me to a chiropractic clinic that I was driving by each day, and it just so happened that I got a good chiropractor. I have used many chiropractors and never had a bad one, but Dr. B by far was the most thorough one I have ever been to. He had worked with games athletes and was a CrossFitter, too, so he could look at me apart from the chiropractic side of it. Because I was new to the area, he was also a great go-to person for other referrals, such as deep-tissue massage therapists. I got myself lined up there, too.

Dr. B became a huge key in my training and imparted so much more on me. He had an annual plan for me to look at over time. He wanted to know how he could take care of my structure to improve it. Many athletes I know do not go to a chiropractor for many reasons. One I would like to address is cost. Many chiropractors have a payment plan if you commit to seeing them for long periods. I had a good experience with one in Redding. For $300 paid up front, you could see him once a week for six months. If you needed him more than once a week, an additional visit was five bucks. I saw him more than once a week on a few occasions, but he never charged me the extra five bucks. My insurance does not cover chiropractic care because I have a huge deductible to meet, and then the chiropractor must be in network, so I need a reduced plan. Dr. B. also offered a substantial discount if I committed and paid in full for a full year. If you don't think being in balance and aligned correctly doesn't make a difference in your health—and therefore your training and competition—you are wrong, my friend, dead wrong. Being aware of your body and what is going on is crucial in performing your best. Dr. B was also performing recovery tests on me with a machine he has that mainly measures heart rate, skin temperature, and a few other things. This would prove to be an excellent tool later.

CHAPTER 12

EQUIPMENT

HAVING GONE THROUGH this CrossFit process and participating and competing in other sports, I have always treated equipment with importance. CrossFit is no different in my book in the quality-equipment department. I started gathering equipment within my first year of CrossFit. I made sure I had a nice gym bag and had it with me at all times, loaded with everything I might need. I say *might* because you never know what you will need or what your buddy next to you might need. Some of the items in my gym bag include lifting shoes; lifting-crossover metcon shoes; my jump ropes (two, in case one breaks); two lifting belts; voodoo floss; a lacrosse ball; knee sleeves; gloves; shin sleeves for rope climbing; chalk; a sweatband; athletic tape; Deep Blue muscle cream; and food consisting of pre-WOD shakes, recovery shakes, and protein bars. I also keep a piece of organic fruit and a small bag of freshly chopped, organic veggies. These are the things you can get into your body quickly.

You have to be able to look at the WOD and know what you need. For example, if the WOD has fifty C2B, then there is a good chance of ripping the hands. I'm going to use the gloves, because I am not going to destroy my hands for several days and lose training time. I always protect my shins now in rope climbing. I have learned my lesson with my battle scars, and I don't need more at this point in my life by being stubborn, prideful, cheap, or just ignorant. I have learned what to carry by experience but also by learning from others, listening to them, and doing what they suggest to avoid unnecessary injuries.

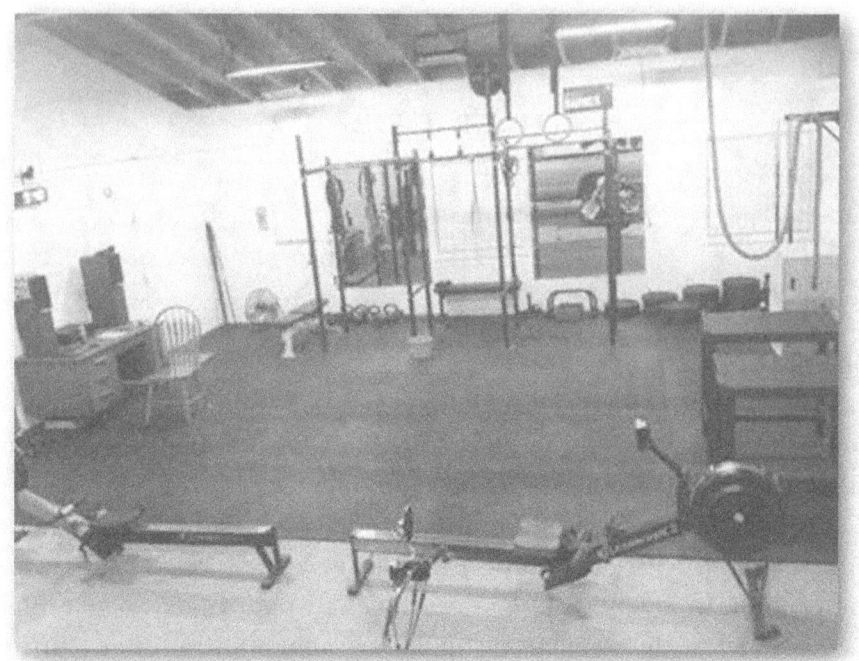

Rodeo Blues CrossFit box equipped with quality equipment.

Lifting shoes are important. I love the stability they provide on the floor. They help with my ROM, which is going to get me bigger numbers. They have raised heels, allowing increased ROM of the ankle, thereby putting me into a deeper squat position. Staying vertical becomes easier, thereby preventing injuries and increasing performance. I always try to talk people into purchasing lifting shoes as soon as possible. It's so simple that it's almost silly. I think most people don't understand the benefits of them or don't want to pay to own them. It has to be a priority. Why not make your training performance a priority and utilize every advantage available so you can be the best you can be? You can get great deals on these shoes nowadays, and you can also buy used ones. I have found some of my equipment at Play It Again Sports and thrift stores, on Craigslist and Amazon, and from friends. Where there is a will, there is a way.

CHAPTER 13

PREPARING AND COMPLETING THE OPEN

THE OPEN CAN be intimidating for many people. Experience and being prepared can eliminate a lot of unnecessary stress and wasted energy. Your prior training should have you well prepared and in your best shape for the five weeks of the open. Have an experienced coach guide you. Listen to your coach, and do what he or she says to the best of your availability. The more experience you have as a CrossFitter, the more you will improve at the open. I was nervous when I did my first CrossFit open in 2013. I definitely lacked experience, but in a way, I think that may have helped me stay calm and productive because I didn't know what to expect. What I disliked the most about the open in 2013 was being such a beginner as a CrossFit athlete. Being from a newer box, we all lacked experience. I repeated all my WODs except one. That's how I made it to the games in 2013—that, combined with being consistent. My coach and I would sit and strategize on what to do differently and how to get a better score on the repeat. The way I "WODed" back then, I exerted a lot more nonproductive work, but because I was in such great shape, I got away with it. We would clean up some of it on the repeat, but form and technique still lacked. Because I had to repeat so many of the WODs, I lost a lot of productive training time. I was always recovering during the open to commit to the next WOD or repeat the previous WOD. Some of those WODs that Dave Castro programmed felt terrible. Each time I repeated a WOD, my score was always better. My drive and my becoming a little more efficient are what attributed to the better scores.

My open in 2014 was not my best by far. Even though I had another year of CrossFit experience in me, and I was a better athlete, programming proved to be more advanced and more competitive than it had been in 2013. I was not ready for it. The programming had a lot more gymnastics in it that year, and that was still my weakest aspect. Moving my own body weight was tough.

I also had put a ton of pressure on myself to perform for my coach because I respected him greatly. I also wanted to perform for my family, friends, and fellow CrossFitters. I felt obligated not to let anybody down because they had invested so much in me, including my sponsor, 321 Apparel.

Again, I had to repeat every WOD except for one. I was quite unprepared during this open. My weaknesses stuck out like a sore thumb. I screwed up right off the bat with C2B. I could do them—but only one at a time, and they faded fast at that rate. Coaches were thinking that they would not ask my age group to do MUPs, but they did, as well as C2B, which are both considered advanced gymnastics moves. I wish I had had the knowledge to understand back then how important it was to relax and enjoy the moments in the open. Have some fun, and be proud of all the improvement, not focusing on the failure. I took every part of it so seriously. It was actually hard to believe I finished up in the open, twenty-first in the world, with all that negativity going on in my mind, as well as some poor repeated scores. That was enough to get me into the masters' qualifying round. I could not place high enough in that round to go to the games without the MUPs under me that year in that age group.

As I look back, the biggest disappointment to me is how hard I was on myself. I didn't realize I was still very much a rookie, and it takes time to mature and gain skills. I had the chance to enjoy the journey, but I chose to be disappointed in my performance instead. I did take that disappointment and turn it into a determined training program for 2015 rather quickly, though. I had read many CrossFit articles, which stated CrossFit athletes don't start to mature in their performance until three years in. This meant 2015 was again going to be my year.

So, going into the open for 2015, I was a totally different athlete, both in mind and in body. My attitude was that I had trained as hard as I possibly could, utilizing all the possible time allotted from the previous open to the present open. I had taken no shortcuts whatsoever. I had diligently worked on my weaknesses. I was working with top coaches in programming, gymnastics, and long-term open experiences, and my recovery and nutrition were dialed in. I was going to remain calm and be present, both physically and mentally, to enjoy every bit of it. It was my journey, and my journey was going to be enjoyable and fun. I deserved this, and I had seen other top athletes enjoy themselves.

I did get through the open with flying colors! I had a great time, and everything felt way better than I had expected. I have to attribute a lot of this success to some things that were added, like the personal programming Coach Jon had done just for me. He knew me better as an athlete than did any other person in CrossFit, and he had the knowledge and skill to program for me. As hard as the workouts were, it was tempting to skip days or do less, but I never did that. I worked as hard as my body could take it each workout. When I would ask Coach Jon why he made my programming so difficult, he would say it was because he knew I could take it, and when the open came, he wanted the open workout to be easy and for me to have fun.

That comment did not make me feel any better as I grinded through those workouts. I am not going to go so far as to say the open workouts were easy, but I would say I could do all the movements proficiently with a nice score, and that was certainly fun. A huge plus was that I was prepared and fit. I did not have to repeat any of the WODs, thus allowing me to recover and stay on track for the masters' qualifying round and games training. Another plus was that I was working in a laid-back box with a laid-back coach. They had a twisted and fun sense of humor. Anybody who knows me knows I have a huge amp about my persona, and mixing that up with stillness was rewarding. You see, I have this work ethic that does not let up, regardless of who is there. I have only one gear naturally, but in the past, I have allowed myself to cease under a certain amount of pressure to perform. I did not know this about myself until I changed environments. Having a calm that could turn into a storm proved to be rewarding for me. Taking a lot of pressure off me allowed me to focus and go into a realm all its own. Coach Ben was excellent at keeping the pressure off me, even off the floor in conversations.

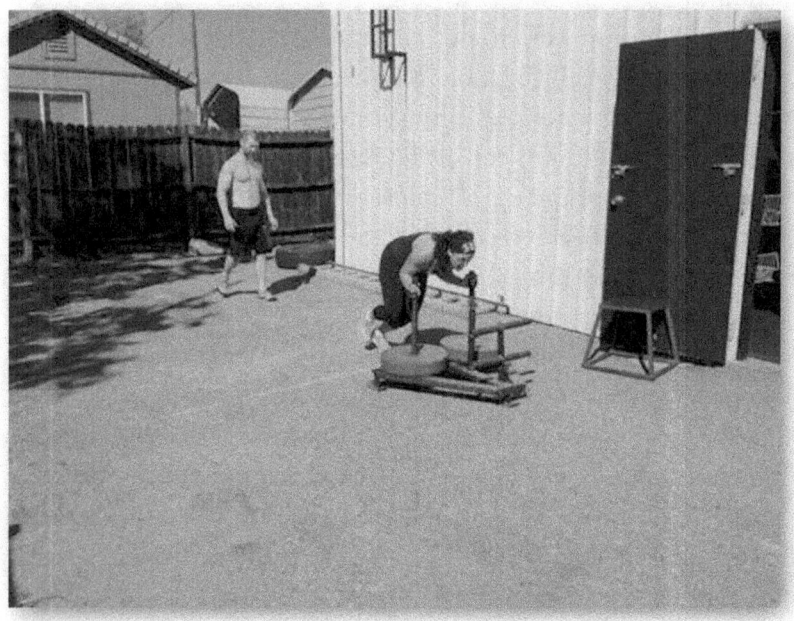

Coach Jon and I working the program before moving to the coast.

My thought process regarding competing in the open was different than in 2013 or 2014. I was focused on the big picture. What does that mean? If you are planning on competing at the games, you cannot go into the open thinking you are going to do whatever you can to get your best score possible. I have done this in the past, and most of the CrossFitters I know have thought or are still thinking along the lines of getting the best score possible at all costs in every one of the five WODs.

It will bite you in the butt sooner or later. First of all, you should have been training and utilizing every opportunity preparing for the open from the last open. Because you are already prepared for the open, you can't possibly be any better at this point, and you have done all the work to the best of your ability. You organize your open WOD around your training schedule. You don't want to lose five weeks of training time that's going to make you the best at regionals or the masters' qualifying round because you are solely committed to the open and are repeating WODs and recovery from each one. Each one of your open WODs should be perfectly executed so you do not have to repeat them. Repeating them not only takes away from productive training days but also increases your opportunity of injuring yourself. Overtraining takes away the opportunity to compete in the masters' qualifying round or regionals and then games. So, having all your training done before the open and being the best you can be before the open can remove those chances of injury by having to do each WOD only once and coming out with a great score the first time out. Recover and then get on to your training before the next WOD arrives.

Part of the perfect execution outside your outstanding training is to be patient. Just because the WOD format has been announced does not mean you have to do the WOD that night. I highly recommend tuning in each time CrossFit announced the WOD and watching it a number of times. You will learn a lot from watching that. The other video that I like to watch is "Rudy" from Outlaw Way. Rudy released a thought process on how to attack the WODs most efficiently. I utilized his methods in 2015 and found him to be spot on. You can also watch other members' WODs before watching yours and learn from their methods, or learn from their mistakes. Just get yourself together, and be ready with proper diet, rest, and equipment. Getting somebody to judge you who has lots of experience is crucial. He or she will know how to set up your equipment in the most proficient manner and help you make decisions. Even the smallest bit of help, like the heel of a lifting shoe, can give you an edge—an edge that can give you a winning score. Be smart, and stay calm. Really, the only time you should have to repeat a WOD is if something goes wrong, such as the timer broke, you were not feeling up to par, or the judge made an error. Repeating them otherwise means you're not ready; in that case, you're not going to the games anyhow.

I was fortunate enough to have the same coach/judge throughout my entire open in 2015, Ben Green. We usually waited a day or two before completing my WOD. By then, he had watched and coached many athletes through it already and had lots of pointers to execute the best of my ability score. He knew how to set everything up to allow the best working environment. It worked every time for me. Several people asked me if I was going to repeat my WOD to get a better score, and I said I was in this for the big picture and mentioned all the reasons why I was not repeating them unless absolutely necessary. People were perplexed by my idea, but I had to look ahead farther than the open at that point to get to the games. I hope it made sense to some, even more so when they saw I qualified for the games.

The combination of my open scores put me in third in the world and first in the United States. I never repeated any of the WODs, and that made a huge difference for me in decreased stress, quicker recovery, and keeping me on track for training for the masters' qualifying round. Having fun and feeling good put me in a position where I was encouraged to help others during the open. I thoroughly enjoyed this. In 2015, CrossFit headquarters required anybody who judged to have a judging certification in order to judge officially. I did want to help my box any way I could and support the other members, so I paid the reasonable fee and took the course online. I was certified before the open. By doing this, I could legally judge in the CrossFit open, and it also gave me a nice training background for judging. The course was not easy to complete. I learned many new things about judging certain movements to bring them to standards. This information also would help me keep my standard up to par.

Doing well in the open validated my admission to compete in the masters' qualifying round. There is about a three-week window between the open and this competition. They take the top two hundred from my age group around the world. This is completely different from the requirements for regionals and from the masters' qualifying rounds of previous years. During this time, I was taking precautions on staying healthy in all ways possible and keeping up with my training. I managed to get a small cold but shook it off by the time the qualifier rolled around, and I lost little training time.

I want to talk about this cold. I see a lot of people coming into the box and training when they are sick and contagious. I saw an articles board that had a rule saying that if you are sick, stay home. I think this is great advice, but also I don't think it can help your training if you are sick. More than likely, it will make you sicker or sick for longer periods. It's important for box owners to keep their boxes clean as well.

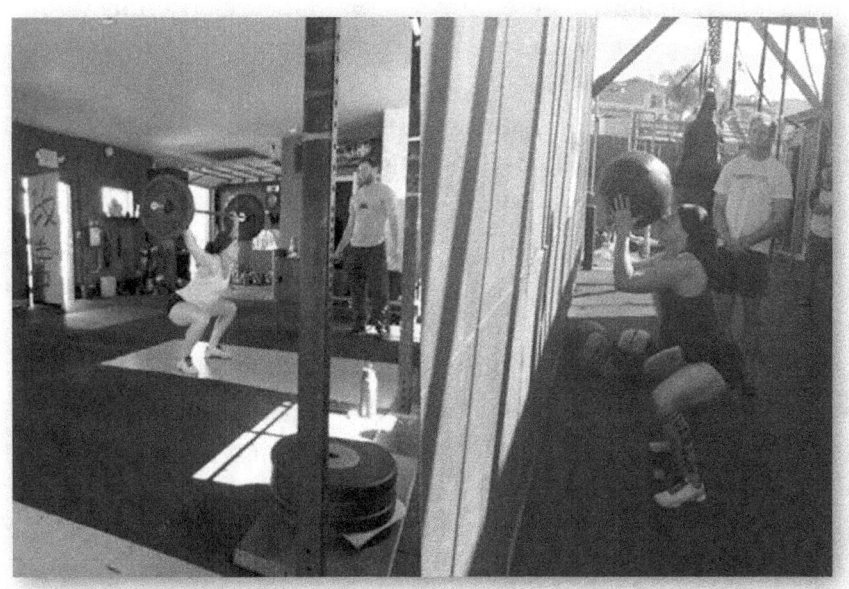

Coach Ben judging me during 2015 CrossFit Open competition.

CHAPTER 14

GETTING THROUGH THE MASTERS' QUALIFIERS OR REGIONALS

EVEN THOUGH I have never competed at the regionals, I think they are similar to the masters' qualifiers in how to prepare for them and get through the process. I also think the masters' qualifying round will eventually be held in a similar fashion to the regionals, as the masters' fields continue to grow rather than stay in a box and be filmed. That is what has been required since 2014. All year long, the training would be cycling through strength programs, including weight and body-weight movements, all the variations of metcons. Utilize and become familiar with any new equipment that Rogue releases and anything else you can think of. Coach Jon was good at racking his brain and programming everything under the sun for me so that I would not get any surprises. You cannot get much training done while competing in the masters' qualifying round because you have four WODs to complete in just five days. This is where recovery is crucial. You have to take the time after each WOD to aid in recovery to prepare for the next in the best possible shape. For me, I was prepared from all the greatly matched programming, doing all the programming work, and having a coach who lined me up properly and efficiently for each WOD and kept me calm. I even won the one-rep-max snatch event and got a PR of 125. (The snatch is an overhead Olympic lift; in 2013, I could not get even one hundred pounds over my head.) Ben helped me out so much. He reminded me of some simple technical advice during the event to secure my win. I do hope I express how grateful I am to these amazing coaches and their dedication toward me. It can make all the difference having these people in your court.

I did have an amazing, supernatural experience that must be remembered. It was the last WOD I was to perform by our order of choice. It was three rounds of rowing, thrusters, and pull-ups. I was hoping for C2B—I had finally mastered them—and I knew they would be coming at the games. So, all these movements were definitely in my wheelhouse, and we were confident this WOD would go very well.

On round three, I started to feel a little strange on the rower and became a little worried. At this point, I started praying to God silently, and I noticed some shadow of a person in my peripheral vision. I tried to ignore it and just pass it off as children playing outside the overhead door, as I wanted to stay focused on the WOD. By now, the shadow became apparent on my left side, and it was behind my coach, Ben. I looked over at him, and Ben looked behind himself to see what I was looking at. This happened three times. On the third time, I looked over there and saw Jesus in a robe. He was pointing and laughing at Ben's purple, high-top tennis shoes. It was a major distraction that allowed me to get through that last round without thinking about any of the pain. They don't call me Crazy Chelle for nothing.

Afterward, I had to share my story with all those athletes who came to watch me do my last WOD. It was an amazing WOD and something I will never forget. I later watched the video, and you can see me looking over at something several times and Ben looking and turning around to see what the heck I kept looking at. At one point, I actually tried to tell him what was going on, but he told me I could tell him later. Good advice! All my combined scores allowed me to place number one in the United States and number three in the world—talk about consistent scores! And I was going to the games just as long as my videos passed their validation process. My coach was not worried about the videos. He said my standards were excellent.

I was worried. My video validation came back approved shortly after, and alas, the final stages of preparing and training for my next trip to the games had arrived. This was a dream come true. I was excited and thankful for all the hard work and strategizing with the programming. It had finally all paid off. This was amazing! I was ready to do more work to prepare to do my best at the games.

CHAPTER 15

PREPARING FOR THE 2015 GAMES

AFTER QUALIFYING FOR the games, I was given a full week to rest mentally and physically. Coach Jon told me to stay active and do things outside the box. It sounded great to me, but it is so hard to stay out of the training mode when you have been training so hard for so long. It is ingrained in you to work hard, and I would feel guilty. But I understood his point, especially for recovery. I would give in to the rest. My training for the games would not be optimal if I did not listen to him.

The other thing that was cropping up with me during rest bouts was depression. My chiropractor credited that to the serotonin drip. Serotonin is a happy chemical we create in the brain and is increased by exercising. When you are exercising for three hours a day, you have a pretty good serotonin drip going on, which can induce euphoria. When that was cut down or went away, I wasn't feeling so great. It was addicting, but I knew I could find other ways to produce it while not exercising or keep my mind busy when it was low. So, I became good at fighting that. When that feeling came about me, which was usually during any extended downtime, I read my Bible. Sometimes, I would go for a walk, find the sun for a few minutes, walk the shores of the beach, walk through a store, go for a nature hike, or text a friend. At times, it was a constant battle.

Dr. B was awesome at letting me share some of my most embarrassing, real moments with him. Rather than passing judgement on me, he would listen to me and help give me ideas on how to combat these types of things that rise up, and he would try to keep me being my best. He was also becoming regular on his recovery testing, as the games training was on in full. He was testing me once a week, looking to make sure I was recovering the best I could. It started out with good scores, which insured I wasn't overtraining and I was recovering from the training. The three recovery tests he ran on me were surface EMG (muscle tone), thermal scanning (temperature regulation), and heart rate variability. The scores from these tests told us how stress was affecting my overall health and well-being.

I wasn't too far along into training for the games when I started getting some bad recovery scores. After I had several poor scores and a few talks with my chiropractor, Coach Jon looked at my food journal and discovered I was lacking calories and complex carbohydrates. I had been sticking with the Paleo diet, but I was not getting enough glycogen according to all the extra work I was doing getting ready for the games. I added another one thousand calories per day and added white rice and white potatoes. When I first started eating these two foods, a surge of energy and happiness came over me. I guess that's why carbs are known as the "happy food." They tasted good, too. But they soon got old, and I was forcing them down. However, it did change my recovery test scores. They improved dramatically and more than likely saved me from an issue that would have cropped up. I never noticed much of a change in my training from day to day, but I felt much better and happier. Sleep was holding steady at ten to twelve hours per night. The amount of sleep required to train like a beast day in and day out is crazy. When I told people how many hours I slept, many could not believe it, and I am sure they thought I was taking some form of a prescription to help me sleep or I had a health issue. I often wondered if training this hard for such long periods would create a health issue in me. It seems like a bit of an extreme most of the time. But it is amazing how much the body can take.

Coach Jon's programming was creative. He was always striving to leave no stones unturned. The programming was never much fun because it was designed for me to get stronger and work on my weaknesses. For example, he knew I was naturally good at long-endurance WODs. He rarely would program them to accommodate my fun. Instead, he would program short metcons. Because I was a bigger athlete with long twitch fiber, short bursts were not my cup of tea. So, we would work hard on those to get as much improvement as possible.

I would find myself lying on the floor after nearly every WOD. Most of the time, I could get right up, but sometimes I was there for a bit. Rarely would Coach Jon program movements that I was very good at. Instead, the metcons would have the movements in them that I needed the most work in. At times, it was so frustrating because I was always working hard to improve them. I had little fun struggling through these short bursts with as much speed as I could put up with. One day, I was talking with Ben about my weaknesses, and he said, "You mean your strengths."

At that moment, I realized that many of my weaknesses were now my strengths. I had conquered them, especially in my age group. That old saying that hard work pays off was culminating for me. I am so hard on myself that having a compliment like that was a reality check and boosted my confidence. You need to surround yourself and work with those types of personalities. I still had a few body-weight movements to conquer—namely, handstand walks and MUPs. The likelihood of them being programmed at the games in my age group was slim, but it was still a possibility. Anyone who is familiar with CrossFit knows Dave Castro can ask for anything.

Another way of looking at the training for gymnastics was that by going through the progressions, I was going to gain ROM and become stronger. The biggest issues with the progressions was to avoid getting injured; extra training on top of heavy training; more training time; working through the pain; and accomplishing them, especially at my age. Progressions are the movements building up to the advanced movement. I had spoken to Ben about them not long after I arrived, and we worked on them from time to time. Yet for some reason, it wasn't clicking or happening. I decided it was time to get a CrossFit person who had gymnastics experience. I still had some time to work on them. I had obtained the CrossFit gymnastics certification in the fall of 2014 when I went to Anchorage but had not taken advantage of what I had learned. I had forgotten most of it. Working with a technical-gymnastics person was going to have many benefits other than learning to achieve a MUP. It was time to make take this MUP thing into my own hands and perform the movement.

CHAPTER 16

ACHIEVING ADVANCED MOVEMENTS

As WITH YOUR nutrition, health, financial planning, or exercise program, you have to be responsible for yourself and make your own choices on what you think is best for you. If things go south, you have no one to blame but yourself, and that's the best route to take.

I had started working on MUPs shortly after I began CrossFit. No proper technical instructions were available for a strict or kipping MUP at the box where I started CrossFit. At the time, I did not know I needed that because I was so new to the sport. It's definitely not something a coach would teach a beginner in CrossFit anyhow. But I would teach certain skills to beginners to prepare them for later, and those skills help them in so many other ways—for example, having tension in their body. Having the technical skills in check decreases risk of injury, teaches body awareness, achieves the correct ROM, improves strength, and allows you to teach or assist others correctly who are trying to get their first MUPs. I also did not have the upper-body strength to perform one, so MUPs were not going to happen. I was also told by several people CrossFit headquarters would not ask a master at my age to do them because injuries are common, especially when you don't have proper training or the strength to complete one. I stayed away from them and focused on getting stronger. Looking back on it, I wish the road to MUPs had been different for me, as I failed to qualify for the games in 2014 because of MUPs. I thought that God had a plan for me, and he sure did.

The MUPs cropped up again in the 2015 masters' qualifying round, and of course I did not get one. The WOD that had the MUPs in it was a triplet (three different moves), and I scored very high on the other two moves, which had a tiebreaker score in it because very few gals my age could do a MUP. So, the outcome of me not being able to do one did not affect my score poorly in that WOD or my overall score. I also noticed most of the gals who got a MUP had poor scores consistently across the board. Only a handful could do MUPs and receive decent scores. I figured those girls who had received the MUPs and scored poorly in the majority of the other WODs had gymnastics backgrounds of some sort. Just a guess. I slid by again, but you know that bothered me. I wasn't happy by any means—even at fifty-five—to be a world-class CrossFit athlete and not have MUPs down. What is the smartest and safest way to achieve an advanced movement? Acquire someone who is reliable, because your time is sparse. That person should specialize in the movement and be a good teacher. If he or she has CrossFit coaching or competing experience, kudos! I started asking around, and my deep-tissue massage therapist and chiropractor both came up with the same name: Siera Lutz.

Contacting her was a pleasant experience. She was delighted to help me, had time to give me, and wanted nothing in return. We started at the beginning of MUP progressions and from nothing but a strict, technical standpoint. The things she taught me all made sense. I could see we wouldn't rush getting this done, and yes, I should have started this type of training back in 2013. But she was hopeful and positive. Even though in the back of my mind I thought the reality of actuality getting a MUP before the games was slim, I could see so many benefits from her practice with me. What an amazing young lady she was. Each week, I was making headway and progressing nicely. I knew I was blessed to have her on team Chelle. These are the type of people you keep on your team and surround yourself with: positive, motivated, and upbeat. I know I keep repeating that, but drama and negativity are out of the question when you are in this type of training. You will need to be able to go to these people and bounce all kinds of stuff off them. How they react and reply can make all the difference. Siera is a coach who was a talented athlete and extremely patient, kind, positive, full of information and experience, and hard working.

Lacking mobility in my shoulders and having a heavy training schedule were the opposing factors that forced me to fail initially. My shoulders were so sore that it was hard to do more MUP work. After much practice and even changing the scheduling practices when I was considered fresh (coming off rest), lack of strength in my back was not allowing me to connect the swing and pull; thus, I couldn't achieve one before the games. Even the accessory pieces I was doing to strengthen that part of my back needed more time to make the gains I needed. It was too late to make it a priority. But we kept at it, meeting usually twice a week, being extra cautious not to injure myself or exhaust myself to the point that it would interfere with my training. Siera was a breath of fresh air. It was nice to have a person to train with me physically, be by my side, and to talk with.

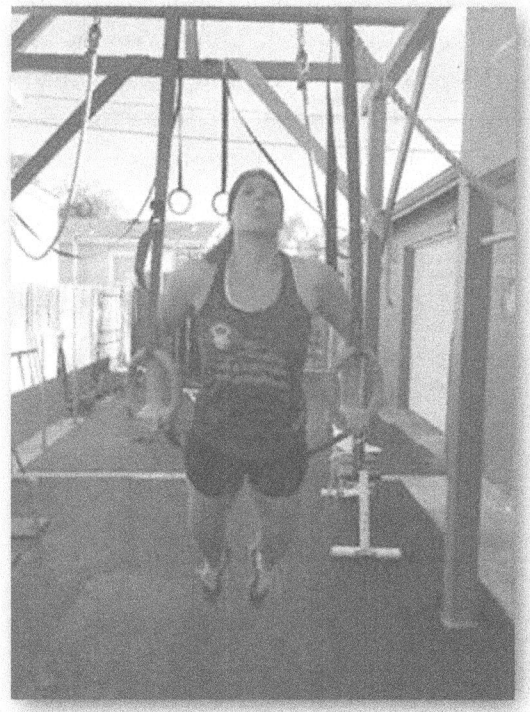

Practicing MUPs through progressions.

The best-case scenario to achieve advanced movements is to allow yourself the time to train technically for them before they are needed and to capitalize on getting the best coaching available to assist you for all the reasons we discussed. If you need to work on your OLY, then you need to find someone who specializes in teaching OLY. That may mean traveling to a different box a few times a week or bringing someone into your box to work with you a few times a week. In 2013, I knew I needed help with my OLY, and I went out and found it. Guess what? I won the snatch event in the masters' qualifying round in 2015. My worst lifting movement became my best. I won that because I worked hard on it and never gave up on it, and it was a two-year process. Coach Jon said we beat that one to death with a stick after I won that event laughing. Was it worth it to me? Absolutely. Do I still work on improving and getting my snatch lift better? I certainly do, and I feel secure in teaching it to others now. I did get my Olympic weight lifting certification in September of 2014 in the state of Washington. The instructors buried me in that course because those lifts are so technical, but I made it through the weekend and earned my certification. Today, it makes sense and all comes together. It can be fun to watch others who are just learning it, for most of them try to do all the same things that all the new lifters do.

CHAPTER 17

COMPETING AT THE GAMES AND MAKING THE PODIUM

DRIVING TO SOUTHERN California to compete at the 2015 games was completely different than in 2013. I was prepared physically and mentally, as well as relaxed and happy. I knew what to expect. I was super excited and could hardly wait to start the competition. The confidence was there because I had taken every step possible to train and recover the best I could possibly do. I had put the time in. I had a ton of support from my current and past CrossFit boxes, my coaches, my recovery peeps, my friends, and my family. It was as if they were depending on me to do a great job, but the pressure was not there, just the love. Even my sponsor, 321 Apparel, was a huge support and told me so many times how proud they were of me. This made me feel so good, as if I had met my part in their contract. In 2013, I had felt different, unprepared, and nervous about the unknown.

It takes several days to make sure you have all the appropriate things packed that you will need. The equipment, clothing, supplements, and food are four of the most important things to pack. Your accommodations in your hotel need to meet your needs. Think of refrigerators, a way to heat your food, and—for goodness sake—a bathtub. If the hotel has a sauna, that could be a bonus, as well as a gym to roll and stretch out in. Make sure the hotel is close to everything you need. Headquarters is good about giving you instructions on everything you will need to do, but traffic could be an issue. You also know you are going to get $5,000 worth of Reebok clothing, gear, and shoes when you check in. In exchange for this gift of clothing and equipment, you are required to wear and use

Reebok items solely while on the field. It's wonderful they do that, but it can be a little difficult. Trying to get used to new clothing in the form of a uniform is something you have to block out. No one wants to break in a new pair of lifters on game day or run sprints in new shoes, so you need to make sure you're wearing Reebok shoes year round, for the most part. That way, you can still wear your current shoes that you have been lifting in or running in. I wish Reebok would put some effort into a good powerlifting shoe. If you take any equipment out on the field that is not Reebok, you must cover the brand name with tape.

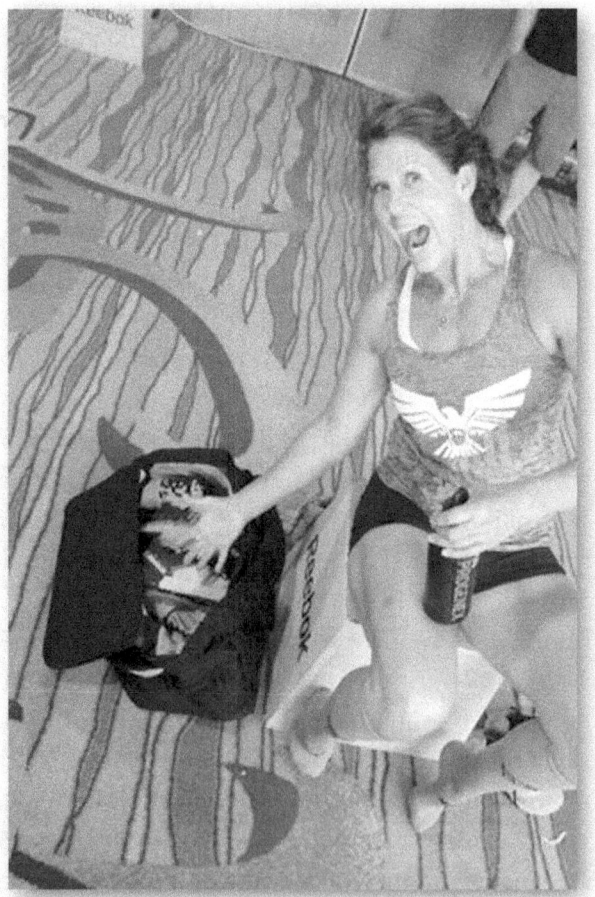

Receiving Reebok shoes and gear for the Games.

To stay on top of my game, I made sure I stayed on top of letters from CrossFit headquarters via e-mail and checking with CrossFit.com several times a day for updates. I felt organized and had a plan on how to stay that way. I had several master athletes ask me what I do about eating at the games. Primarily, we try to pack the majority of our food, thereby having highly nutritious foods available at all times and reducing the risk of getting sick. I also like to eat the same things almost every day. I definitely don't want to change my food plan while at the games. My body is used to well-planned nutrition. I don't want to be driving around in the early morning and late afternoon trying to find nutritious or particular foods. The traffic is hectic in Southern California, so wasting time driving around getting food is increasing your chance of an accident. Getting sick or losing recovery time does not make sense to me. Going out for food is expensive, too, and you don't know what you are getting into. The food might not be fresh, so packing the majority of my food was a necessity. It's part of a winning team and being organized. As I have said so many times, training and competing at a world level is a full-time job. I am not going to turn it into a second part-time job. Being efficient and organized is one big WOD.

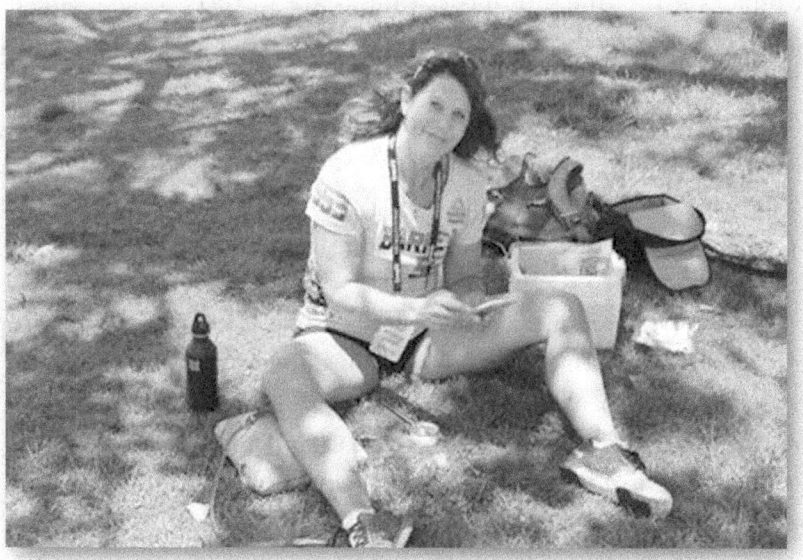

Nutrition break and checking social media.

CrossFit headquarters released all the masters' WODs except the finals. Many days before it was time to depart, it gave me a chance to set up every WOD and practice it at least once and still recover with rest. This was awesome. In previous years, they have not done this. I think they should also release the masters' qualifying round WODs early, too, as they do for the regional athletes. They get quite a lot of time to practice those WODs for regionals. Why shouldn't the masters get the same opportunities?

I felt good about every WOD. Ben was awesome at helping and coaching me through them. He was worried about one WOD where we were required to squat snatch, and sprint. He was nervous about me sprinting but did not share that with me at that point. It is great: you get to practice these WODs and know what they are before you arrive. As mentioned previously, I did not have that chance in 2013, and much anticipation and worry was running through me. Instead, CrossFit headquarters released only a few of them before most people departed to Southern California. There was not enough time to practice them before the games. Those girls who lived in Southern California may have had a little time, but most athletes are in rest mode at this point. It still would be different doing them on the field with these gals, but it definitely rid much of my anxiety by knowing some of the unknown and having the opportunity to complete them and organize most efficiently. It also organizes you as to what equipment you will or possibly need, so it gets packed in your suitcase for sure. It was game changing to practice those WODs, every one of them, yes! It instilled so much confidence in me.

It's important to have a coach with you at the games, as well as a partner. I was blessed with both of my coaches, Jon and Ben, being there and supporting me. Coach Jon looked bigger than life in the stands. Coach Ben was with me before WODs for warming up and keeping me calm and also in the area where we rested. He even took extra time to cook and bring me extra food. He was also good about texting me about staying upbeat and keeping me on track with my timelines for warm-ups, recovery, and food. He helped fulfill my success at the games in so many ways. I am so grateful for having him in my life and being part of the 2015 CrossFit games. As with Coach Rich and me in 2013, no one can ever take those moments away from me. I'm so blessed! These types of memories are priceless.

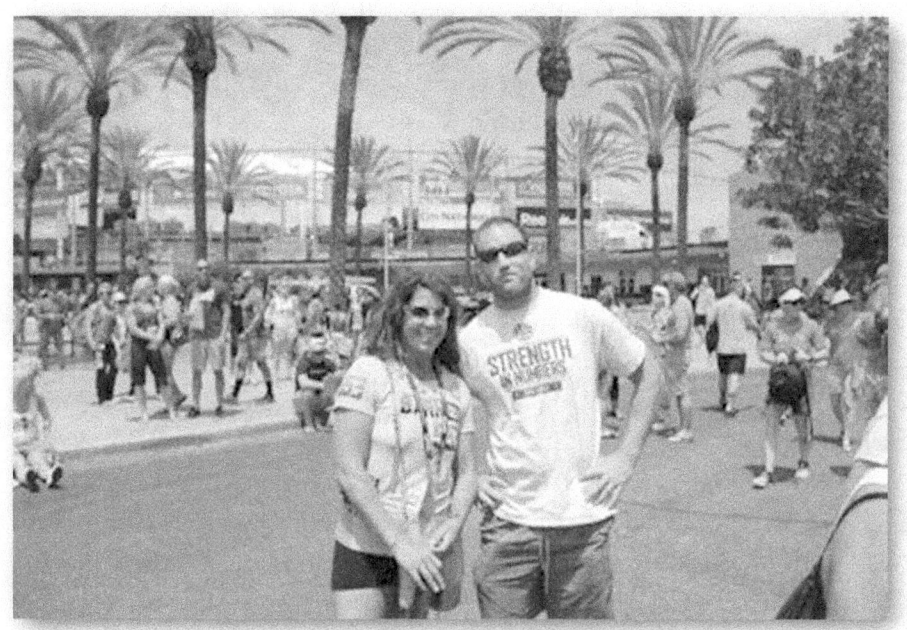

Ben and I attending our Crossfit Games meeting.

My husband was and still is my biggest asset. He certainly made my life much easier by training and supporting me through the games. He was praying for me and with me, eating all the same food I did, training with me, going to bed early, getting up early on his days off from work, supporting and helping pay for my recovery methods, and being my bodyguard at the games. Bodyguard? Well, he designed and set up a rigid schedule at the games and made sure we stuck to it. It can be easy to get sidetracked at the games, as you run into old friends you have not seen in a while. You have friends and family who have come a long way to watch you compete at the games, and they want to visit and eat with you, but you cannot. There will have to be time for that later. Using your time efficiently will help aid you in gaining a winning edge. My husband made sure we were back to the hotel by a certain time after the WODs were completed, and then we would start the recovery processes and get the calories in. Then, it was off to bed—no visitors, no phone calls, no e-mails, and little social media. I was fortunate to be able to fall asleep early and sleep through the night every night. The confidence was there to allow just that, because I did not sleep well in 2013. CrossFit required us to check in early every day between 6:15 a.m. and 6:45 a.m. That was a crazy early time, requiring me to rise at 4:30 a.m. to prepare to be there by 6:15 a.m. I never had any incidents like traffic jams or oversleeping, and I made it on time each day. The schedules we designed paid off and worked well. The organization you commit to must cross over in all areas. My husband was a huge part of my success in both 2013 and 2015. His actions spoke louder than his words, and I could not have done so well without him.

I loved being on the field and competing with the other female athletes. This age group of women was engaging and supportive of one another; it was different than in 2013, when I had been a dark horse. I had popped out of nowhere, and no one knew me, as far as the other girls competing were concerned. The majority of them were returning three or four times. But in 2015, I felt very welcomed and well taken care of. Lots of people were complaining about the heat and humidity. Headquarters provided us with a nice, big building that had air-conditioning, healthy snacks, and good water. They also provided us with lots of people to help us recover, first aid, and ice baths. The climate didn't bother me mentally at all. I was staying hydrated, supplementing, and consuming calories.

Now, eating was very hard. With all the excitement of being there, and maybe some anxiety, my appetite was suppressed, to say the least.

But I was able to force-feed myself, and my husband constantly reminded me to eat and drink, as did I. As hard as it is to eat during this time, it is a must. The fluids were extremely important, as I found out on day one. Every morning, we had a mandatory meeting where CrossFit headquarters went over all the standards with their head judges. It was quite a time-consuming ordeal, lining us all up, marching us down to the field bleachers, and then having the meeting. On the first day, I left my water bottle in our recovery area, thinking I would be gone for only a short period. I was gone too long, and I cramped pretty good in my midsection during the day. It actually made me sore in my core. I figured out quickly that the fluids had to go in constantly. I could not go an hour without taking in a lot. Just by missing that eight ounces, it hurt me physically. I started drinking water as soon as I rose from bed each morning and did not stop until it was time for bed. And if I had to get up in the night for any reason, I made sure I drank water, too.

The time of day that headquarters picked for us to compete in could not have been better, in my opinion. Most of our WODs were done while the temperatures were still decent. I thank Dave Castro for that. I felt good about the weather. It didn't seem to bother me mentally, for I was so focused and ready. This could be dangerous, because you need to pay attention to the heat and humidity, even if your mind suggests differently. Get out of the sun as soon as possible, drink as much fluid as needed, keep your electrolytes balanced, wear proper attire, and get your body cooled. This is where your tribe can be of great help, reminding you in case you get distracted. Make a checklist for them to go over as they check on you periodically. Our rest area was set up on the grass and with a tent cover away from the general population. They called it Tent City.

The first WOD was a bit nerve racking. You're getting settled in, trying to find your way, focusing, figuring out the field and the directions of the WODs, understanding what the judges want, and figuring out the equipment. My first WOD, I believe, was my worst placing. I placed ninth, and this was an easy one for me, but I was playing around out there. Once that WOD was over, I felt like myself for the rest of the competition. The one thing that bothered me on the first WOD was that the glute-hamstring-developer machine was very slick, and I had a hard time getting on and off it. I felt as if I were going to fall. Once I got on, pumping out the reps was not an issue, and neither was any other part of the WOD. This kind of stuff happens; you just don't have much control of it. Did I have that type of trouble on the glute-hamstring developer at home? Absolutely not. Did I let my results for that WOD affect me negatively? Hell no! Every WOD was exciting, and I had a lot of fun doing each of them.

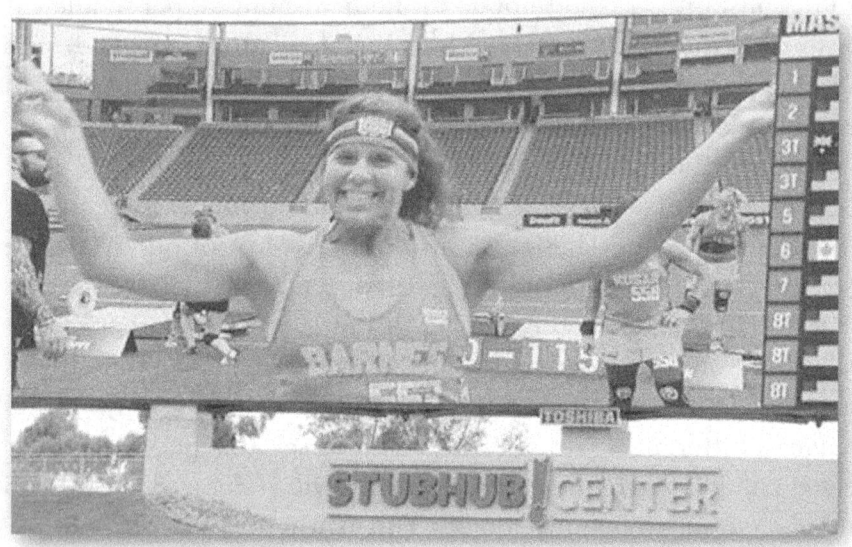

On the big screen after winning WOD two, redeeming myself after WOD 1.

I actually did pretty well and consistent throughout all the WODs. On one WOD, I placed higher than what the scoreboard reported, and part of my team caught it and told me. You have only a certain amount of time after a WOD is completed to appeal it. I had to head back down the tunnel, find a head judge, and fill out the paperwork. I was not down there long, and Coach Ben showed up to support me and help me with the appeal. But he was not allowed in the tunnel, and several of the security guards were after him. The head judge released the security guards and told Coach Ben he could stay and help with the appeal. We won the appeal, and I was awarded my true score.

For some reason, the judge hadn't completed my scorecard correctly. The WOD had a capped time on it, and I had just about finished it. Yet on my scorecard, the judge had me scored back at about three-quarters of the way through the event, not nearly finishing it. When the head judge approached him on it, he recalled exactly where I finished, and our stories matched. He gave me the correct score. If my team had not seen this, it could have been a disaster overall finish for me. Again, I cannot express how important it is to have a team. Having Coach Ben reacting so quickly and supporting me by helping me with the appeal was grounding as an athlete. I was thankful that it was caught and that the appeal process worked out fine. Later, I ran into that judge at one of the early morning standard WOD meetings, and he came over to me and apologized. He said he had no idea how that had happened, other than the fact he had been tired, hungry, and thirsty. I thanked him and was super happy he recalled my actual finishing place. I also thanked him for volunteering his time to judge. He really was a good judge; it had been a mix-up on his part while filling out his paperwork.

In the past, the masters were competing in parking lots, and the masters were then moved to the track and then on to the soccer stadium for 2015. It was neat competing in that stadium. It felt first class all the way. I am grateful to have had the opportunity to compete on both track and field, as well as at the soccer stadium in both my performances in 2013 and 2015. It felt professional, and things have been upgraded for the masters each year. Everything was run so smoothly, and there was so much staff help. It cannot be an easy task to put the games on. CrossFit headquarters did a great job running the masters through their competitions. When things run well like this, it takes a lot of pressure off the athletes. When you are prepared and organized, you take a lot of pressure off yourself.

Only one gal in my group did not return on day two. The whole experience for her was way too overwhelming, and she folded and had to bow out. I felt bad for her because she came from a foreign country. She traveled a long way to have that happen to her.

The only WOD that was not preannounced—meaning we did not know what it was or have a chance to practice it—was the finals WOD. I placed high enough to make it to the finals. My placing had secured me into a third-place podium finish regardless of what happened during the finals. But if I won it, I had a good chance of moving into second or maybe first place! What did that mean to me? More money and a higher-placing medal. I did want it, and I thought for sure I could do it because I was very good at the two movements in it and had worked hard at them. It was squat snatch and ring dips. Unfortunately for me, I had a judge who did not care for my ring dips and also had a few issues with my squat snatches. Once I figured out what she required, I did what she asked, resulting in a fifth-place finish in the finals WOD. I maintained a third-place podium finish. I was beyond myself with happiness because a podium finish was fine with me and a dream come true, along with making it back to the CrossFit Games. I had no disappointments. My people were all positive and uplifting in that finish. We had accomplished what we came for.

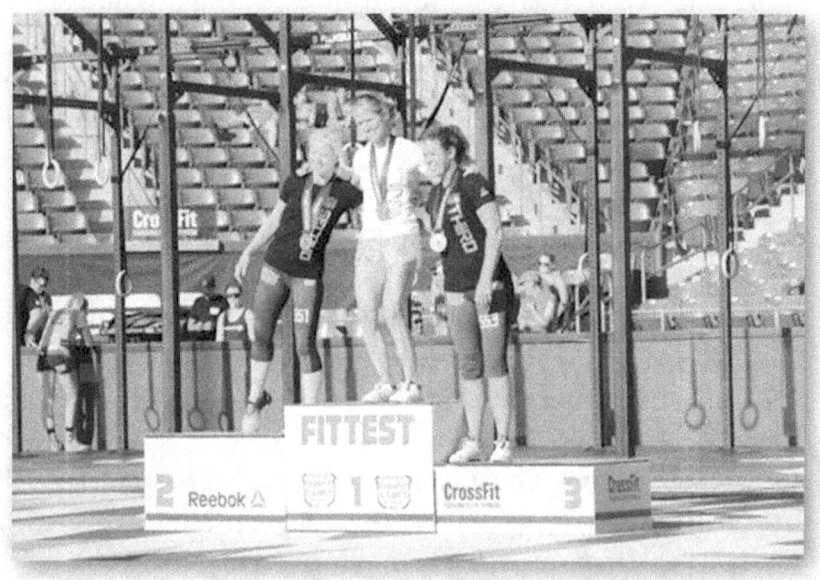

Like I said, "we have accomplished what we came for"!

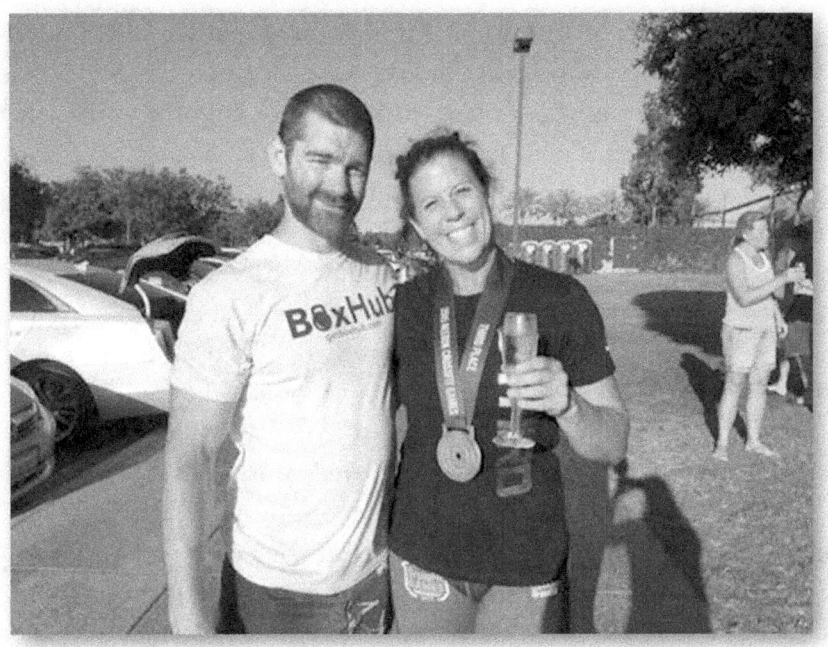

Jon and I celebrating after the 2015 CrossFit Games.

Shortly after completing the WOD, the top three of us were taken from the outside of the tunnel to drug testing. We were escorted by CrossFit personnel. Our identifications were required, which meant we had to get them from our cars or send somebody after them. I understand the process of drug testing, but I didn't like the way it was handled. I was sweaty wet, tired, thirsty, and hungry. We had to wait for the identifications, and then we were taken to the medical team to perform the drug tests by the personnel. We had just been on the tennis courts competing on a ground cover of 120 degrees, and most of us were dehydrated at this point. So, with all that, and with someone I had never met before standing over me, watching and waiting for me to urinate, things did not go over well. I wish they could have just drawn blood, or I wish I could have been better prepared. I could have practiced urinating in a cup while a stranger was watching me.

Seriously, though. I was with the medical team and drank all the water I was allotted and still could not pee for two hours. My friends and family were waiting for me, and some got tired of waiting to hug and congratulate me and left to head home. That was upsetting. The medical team released me to go to the awards ceremony, and then they required me to come straight back to perform the drug test. Of course, as soon as I got to the awards ceremony, I had to urinate. I had the worst full-bladder feeling. I asked a head judge if I could be excused to go back to drug testing, and he told me no! The awards ceremony was hideously painful. I did not enjoy any part of it. All I could think about was getting to the toilet and peeing in front of whomever to get some relief. Once the ceremony was over, I tried running to the area without peeing on myself. I about busted that door down and took cuts in front of everyone, pretty much yelling with rude behavior. There I was, peeing in front of that stranger, and she had me stop halfway so I wouldn't overfill the cup. Oh my gosh, really. I thought I was going to explode. I submitted my urine and was told it was almost too diluted but testable, thank goodness.

So, don't be prepared only to WOD; be prepared for the rituals of drug testing if you have any shot of making the podium. It was an awful experience for me because I was unprepared. Those who had been tested before and knew they would be tested were in and out of there in no time. You have to be secure enough to urinate in front of a stranger while under pressure and tired, hungry, and excited about making the podium, and your water content in your body has to be just right. You can't be dehydrated because then you cannot urinate, and you cannot have had too much water because it dilutes the urine. These were the things I was not prepared for at the games. By the time I got through drug testing twice and the podium appearance, nearly all my family and friends had left. You can let them know the procedure in the future, and they won't stick around and wait for you because, more than likely, you won't be coming out for a while.

I want to talk a little more about drug testing. It took about six to eight weeks for CrossFit headquarters to process the drug test and send out our results. Once that occurred, they mailed out a memento coin and our prize money. Not long after that, I received a letter from CrossFit headquarters stating I would be placed on a random drug-testing policy starting within the next quarter. I was required to fill out paperwork and send it in as to where I would be for the next quarter at all times. If you were going to travel or be anywhere else than what you stated on your paperwork, it was your responsibility to let them know. Every quarter, they send out new paperwork to submit. Failing to comply with any of this is immediate suspension. To this date, I have been on this random drug-testing schedule for a year and one-quarter. I have never been contacted for a random test. I also did not compete in the open in 2016, and I am still on the random drug-testing schedule, so I am not sure if this program is really working for them. However, I do appreciate the fact that they appear to be trying to keep the performance enhancements and other illegal drugs out. It is important to pull out that rule book and read through it at least once. Reading the drug-testing-policy section is a good idea, for the list of illegal drugs is very long, and some of them can easily be in the form of supplements. If I am taking a supplement that has one of the ingredients in it that is on the list and I test positive for it, it is my fault, and no one else is to blame.

CHAPTER 18

DECONDITIONING AND INJURIES

THIS CAN BE a tough time for anyone who has been in some intense training for a long period. For me, the period was 2014 and through 2015 up through the games. It was amazing that I had gotten through all this hardcore training without an injury. I had taken all the precautionary methods I knew to prevent one. I had a few issues crop up but nothing that amounted to anything serious. Everyone around me was telling me to take some time off. Believe me, I wanted to. I was burned out on CrossFit—mainly from the training, not the people or regular one-hour classes, but from the high-intensity volume load. I was also fed up with training alone.

The consensus was that I would take a month off. I feared the worst—namely, that I would fall into a depressive state of mind without all the serotonin surging through me. Many had warned me of this depressive feeling coming in after the games during deconditioning. I didn't have a set plan on how to decondition; I was simply to take some much-earned time off.

I did just that. I'm a pretty active person, so I wasn't lying around on the couch. But I was not Cross Fitting. I was also regularly enjoying some food and drinks that were not in my diet before the games. I was feeling good mentally and enjoying having the time off.

Two weeks had barely gone by, and the craving of going back to exercise was creeping back in. I missed my coach, my peeps, and the box itself, too. I misunderstood my husband because I thought I had asked him how much time off he wanted to take, and two weeks was what we had agreed on. I was later told that my husband didn't say that.

We should have stuck with the month. But after two weeks off, there we were, back at the gym and doing a regular one-hour CrossFit class. That was easy compared with what we had been doing. It was fun not being in a full-blown competitive mode and walking out of there after just an hour, feeling refreshed and good! It was good to be having fun again with everyone.

We had gone in one Saturday morning to WOD, and I think we had been back at it several times after my rest period. This particular morning, the first part of the WOD was ten twenty-five-meter sprints every thirty seconds. I had never seen these programmed in before or done them. As my husband and I were warming up and preparing for the 9:30 a.m. class to start, I recalled several injury warnings regarding sprints. I was inclined to warn the other athletes to make sure they were good and warmed up. I warned them about not running full speed and that twenty-five-meter sprints were really short, which meant needing to accelerate and then having to shut it down. I was thinking many of the athletes might be tired that day from working all week. Maybe they hadn't been following the best diet and had had drinks the night before because it was Saturday morning. Maybe they hadn't had a full night's sleep, or maybe even some were dehydrated.

I felt awkward, as if I were stepping on the coach's toes that day by giving my advice. As it turns out, that advice was for me. We were running the sprints, and we had just completed sprint number eight when I felt my left hamstring and glute tighten. I grabbed it and massaged it a little. I told my husband about it. I had never had anything tighten up like that before, so I had no clue of what was about to happen. We were allotted only thirty seconds to rest, so I didn't have much time to think about it or realize what was going on. I took off on sprint nine at full speed. Halfway through, my left leg just quit, and I tumbled to the ground. Then, I bounced back up, and my left leg went down again. This time, it did not come back up. It was over for me. Everyone was in shock. One guy thought I had been shot by a gun because of the way I had fallen down. I told them to go on and finish, and I went back into the box and hopped onto the assault bike. I slowly started to spin to try to figure out what had happened. I did not have any pain initially, just a misfire of a large-muscle group. When taking steps, I was not sure if my left leg was going to give way.

We got home, and that night the edema started to set in. Then, the pain came. I was planning not to take anything, but because the swelling came in rapidly, I felt I needed to reduce that as quickly as possible, so I started Advil. By Tuesday, my leg was black and blue. I made an appointment with my chiropractor, who in turn convinced me to seek physical therapy for various reasons. That required an orthopedic visit. I was able to get in and see a doctor that week, and he diagnosed me with a third-degree tear of the belly of the hamstring. He told me I would be back to normal in eight to twelve weeks tops. He then sent me off, not even requesting a follow-up appointment or any further testing. He also gave me the order for physical therapy once I asked for it. He stated that he had never seen anyone bleed as I had. The blood was pooled all the way from my butt crease to the back of my ankle—hence, it was very black and blue. It looked as if someone had taken a baseball bat to me. Gravity is what pulls the blood down. Yet I had little pain. I asked him if it was OK to stay as active as possible and resume upper-body workouts, and he stated that that's exactly what he would do—no crutches, no drugs, and stay active. He was a very fit surgeon. I did tell him my background and that I had been named the fittest woman in the United States in my age group.

I resumed upper-body workouts and tried to stay as fit and positive as possible, all while attending physical therapy several times a week. I know most people would have been on crutches and painkillers, confined to the couch. That is not me and not a healthy way to heal, in my opinion. That's a great way to get and stay depressed. Even though the orthopedic surgeon did not know me personally, he had seen enough of his injured athletes become depressed and did warn me about that. As a CrossFit athlete, I knew it was important to stay connected with my box and the other athletes and to stay as fit as I could during this long period of healing. I needed their support, and the easiest way to get that was to go and participate in a modified version of their workouts. Some thought I was insane for showing up to workouts. They wondered if I had seen a doctor at all, and if so, was I doing what he had told me to do? I think the key is to be smart about it and not jeopardize the injured area more. I also think it's important to stay connected with your CrossFit box and be a good role model, even though you're injured or cannot work out for some reason for an extended period.

I did everything the doctor told me to do, including the physical therapy. Although the injury felt better, it seemed as if I had reached a peak with it, and it was not getting any better after about week eight. For example, when I was jogging, I thought part of it was not firing. I could not get any speed out of it. Sometimes, I thought my leg would give way or not be there, as when I was sprinting and the injury occurred. I was also starting to exhibit some tingling and numbness on that injured left side. I tried to stay positive and thought I was taking longer to heal because I was older.

Rapidly approaching twelve weeks after the injury, I knew things were not right, so I called and made a follow-up appointment with the orthopedic surgeon. I also had a discussion with my physical therapist and told her I was putting the therapy on hold until I met with the orthopedic surgeon. Things were not right; even though there was a lot of improvement, it had peaked. I felt something was not right with the doctor I was seeing, either. Even though he was referred to me by my chiropractor and had been on practice as an orthopedic surgeon for a long time, I was nervous about him.

This time, he told me the injury was at the second insertion point of those three hamstring tendons behind my knee. He thought maybe I had detached at that second point by tearing the muscle off, not the tendon. That wouldn't be good because muscle doesn't suture well. He said he had not seen an injury like that for fifteen years.

"But let's be sure and get an MRI," he said.

Get an MRI? Why hadn't that been done already? I agreed with him wholeheartedly. This is where a second opinion could have benefited me greatly. Even though I was unaware that the correct procedure would be to get an MRI, a second and third doctor might have requested that as part of their normal practices.

It took over several weeks to get an MRI scheduled and to get back in to have him read it to me. Once an MRI has been completed, the results go directly to the doctor that day, so the physician has plenty of time to review the report and look at the MRI before the patient's arrival.

Because I was having such negative feelings about the surgeon, I brought my husband along. Once we got into the doctor's exam room and he arrived, I was saddened to learn he had not reviewed it, and he had a hard time loading it into his laptop. Plus, the sun was streaming through the windows and shining on his laptop screen, impeding the clarity of the MRI. I could barely maintain my composure. A full report that he had not read was folded and attached to the DVD. To my dismay, the MRI showed a full detachment of all three tendons from the first insertion point at the butt crease. I nearly passed out when he told me the news. He then stated that this type of injury—since I did not have surgery within the first fifteen days of injury—was way out of his league, and he was going to have to refer me out. He said he would call me later because he needed to find a referral for me. I could not believe what I was hearing. I left his office in shock, wondering if I would ever be able to compete in CrossFit again. What would my quality of life be like in the future? I could not understand why an MRI hadn't been done in the beginning. I started to beat myself up for choosing this doctor, waiting so long to make a second appointment with him, not getting a second opinion right away, and the list goes on. By the time I got to my car, I remembered that God never fails me, and he has a plan. The calm arrived, and I knew I would get through this. I had to rely on him and not panic.

At about 8:30 p.m., I received a very nice call from the doctor telling me that he had a referral set up for me in Santa Monica. He also told me that in the future, he would request all his patients have an MRI for this type of injury. I told him I was glad my mishap would provide a better health care standard for his future patients in a similar circumstance. He told me to call the referred surgeon. The following day, the new doctor and I connected and set up a consult. My husband and I were in his office within a few short days.

Our first consult was pleasing in some senses and scary in others. I did like the fact that his office was full of framed, signed jerseys from high-caliber athletes who ranged from professionals to Olympians. That told me this man knew what he was doing, and he was obviously trusted. The differences in the two doctors' demeanors were like night and day. This one was far more patient, and I did not feel as if I were going through an assembly line. My husband and I had a ton of questions for him, and he answered every one. He palpated me as the other doctor had done several times, and within seconds he found the "stump," as he called it, where all three tendons were hanging out halfway down the back of my hamstring. Once I explained to him I was getting tingling and numbness in that leg, he told me the tendons had most likely wrapped themselves around my sciatica nerve. Great. I was starting to wonder what my quality of life would be like with this leg again. The doctor was positive with me, but he was also honest and said this surgery had no guarantees. It would be difficult to perform because so much time had passed since the detachment. The tendons were no longer stretched and attached to my butt bone; they were shortening themselves and traveling down my hamstring and attaching themselves to—or should I say wrapping themselves around—my sciatica nerve, about the size of a golf ball. I saw this surgeon in mid-November, and the surgery was scheduled that day for December 8, which was the soonest the surgeons could work me in. The injury had occurred on August 6. If anything became available earlier, they would fit me in. Regardless, I was off on a mission to get my preops done as quickly as possible in case they did take me earlier. Because of my age, I was required to get a chest x-ray, an EKG, and blood tests. All these tests came back excellent, which was going to enhance my healing stage. Even though I was injured, I was healthy. If I were smart and obedient, I might have a chance to have a full recovery.

I was eager to get the surgery and also was enjoying walking with two legs and having some freedom. My new surgeon told me I would be on complete bed rest for two weeks and house arrest for another two following the surgery. It would be a good six months before I was back to normal, if the surgery were successful. I was scared. I have never had an injury before that amounted to anything serious, and I had never had a health issue that required surgery, so this was a first at age fifty-five. I knew I was in good health, and the preops revealed that as well, but it was still nerve racking to be still for so long. I would have on a knee-leg brace dialed to ninety degrees, too. This meant one bent leg to sleep on. I kept thinking I should use the time to write the book I had been wanting to write for a few years about health and CrossFit. Actually, ever since I had been a teenager, I had wanted to write a book. I also knew that my relationship with Christ was about to get a whole lot closer. I knew that everything that was happening in my life was ordained by him and that I could get through this through him. That was my peace. I also realized I was going to be able to add an injury chapter to my book with firsthand experience. I was finding the positive in the negative and rolling with it. Yep, I can do this.

So, at this point, I have to confess that I was injured because I did not follow my own advice. I had so much pride and competitiveness in me that morning that we were running twenty-five-meter sprints, and I had turned my training to full heat, running as fast as I could against a twenty-one-year-old ex-marine. Come on. Think about that. How silly is it that I thought I had a chance at beating him in sprinting? He was fit, too. Triple all that with my having no professional experience in running sprints and coming off two years of full-time training. It was a bomb ready to explode. Well, in my mind, I had a shot at it, and I pushed the envelope for sure. I was no longer bulletproof, and now I was going to pay the price for making a poor choice. I had no one to blame but myself. I had a whole different outlook on life, and things were put into perspective very quickly for me that day. The guilt was overwhelming, and I felt like I was a poor role model. I pray that the athletes there that day learned a lot from my foolish mistake. Would taking a month off, as what had been recommended, have prevented this wreck of an injury? I certainly would have missed the sprints that day. Would that have been enough to avoid it? Was there already an injury there, lurking, coming down the pike at some point? About three years earlier, I had been doing high kicks in a dance class and had heard a snap inside that left leg. I think one tendon may have come off or torn at that point there. I had been sore for only a few days and returned to normal dance and lifting. I had never thought another thing about it until this new injury.

I could continue to beat myself up and ask foolish questions, but I didn't see how that would pay off for anyone. I truly believe everything happens for a reason, and I had to find the positive in it and learn, share, and move on. As a coach, I am now more prepared to season my athletes better. Will they listen to me? Some will, and some won't, but just having the opportunity to change the life of one person is enough for me. This is where that quote comes in again: we have to be responsible for our own fitness, and that includes injuries now! Without this injury, I would have never written this chapter, and I would not have had the knowledge to teach others what I learned from the experience.

The surgery was completed on December 8, 2015. What was to take an hour and a half turned into nearly a four-hour surgery, completed by not one surgeon but two. My poor husband was on pins and needles. When the head surgeon came out, he told my husband that if had it not been me, he would have stopped and not gone after my three tendons. I mean, I appreciate who I am, and I am grateful that he wanted to take a chance and go after it, but my heart cannot help but ache over the fact that another fifty-five-year-old grandmother might not have been so blessed to have the surgeon tackle it. She would have ended up living with a leg that had injured muscles, and she would have lived her life in tingling and numbness. I suppose the injury would have worsened over time as well. But then what are the chances of a fifty-five-year-old grandma tearing off her tendons from her butt bone, all while doing twenty-five-meter sprints and then being misdiagnosed? I know it was the first time the surgeons had seen an injury that had gone so long without surgery; the tendons were so far retracted down the back of my leg that he had to make both a vertical and horizontal incision far larger than normal to try to reach them. Normally, it's a small incision horizontally along the butt crease, which you cannot see, for the most part. Even after that, he could barely reach them. So, now I have a lovely battle wound three times larger than what it should have been. Way too much time had passed to make the surgery simple. Once he was able to get the tendons, he had to spend time removing them off my sciatica nerve in the ball they had formed and removed scar tissue. He was hoping that all three tendons would cooperate, and he could stretch them back to the butt bone, but too much time had passed, and he could bring up only one naturally. The other two were attached to other parts of my body, and cadaver material was used to reattach to them to the butt bone. The problem is that cadaver material is not as pliable or as strong as our own tendon material.

Once I woke up from the surgery, my husband had told me it had gone well but had been very difficult, and I would have to take far more rest and care than he had anticipated. I would need to take the maximum amount of pain medications and stay on them for a good two to three weeks, or I would be in a lot of pain. That information was a little hard to digest, but I was pleased the ordeal was over—at least the surgery part. The worst part was having a leg brace on that was set at ninety degrees and trying to wake up from all the anesthesia and the pain medications. I quickly adjusted to the leg brace and understood the necessity of it. It was protecting those tendons from being ripped back off the butt bone. You see, it takes thirty days for those tendons to start to lie down and attach themselves naturally. In the meantime, they were laid down with biodegradable screws.

I made it through that first night and was able to get some decent rest. My husband woke me every four hours so I could ingest a heavy dose of pain medications and a few other medications that helped keep the chances of blood clotting down and infection out. It's also important to focus on detoxing after any surgery. The next morning, we were back in the doctor's office for my first post surgery appointment before we left Santa Monica to return home. The doctor told me that I had made it through the night without ripping it all out, yet he worried I might fall and tear it back off the bone. He reminded me again that it takes thirty days for those tendons to lie back down and attach themselves, so it was up to me and the screws. Another thing he pointed out was blood clots. He was worried about the long car ride home. He asked me to pump my feet as often as possible while sitting in the car and to make a few stops and get out and stretch. I took him seriously. I promised I would obey him and do my best.

I think being older was helpful because it made me realize how serious this was. I was afraid that I could easily screw things up, irreparably this time. I knew I had to be on my best behavior, and I also knew I was going to work this goal through Jesus. That's exactly what happened. I would be in bed recuperating, but I would be writing my first book! The thought of being able to change someone's life for the better through my book was inspiring to me. If I could be a role model for just one person, that whole book would be worth it. I finally was slowed down long enough to take the time to write. What a great way to take something negative and turn it around into something positive.

Jesus provided me with all the mental aptitude I needed to stay dialed in with him and do what was right for my body and him. It became apparent that I was to try to complete this book. He provided all the skills and confidence I needed to get started on it, all while I was on bed rest.

Never once was I restless to get off bed rest or leave the house. I was not bored, and I felt totally fulfilled as I lay rested and healing. If you know me well, you surely understand what a miracle that was, because I do not sit. My days start with, "How much can I get done before bedtime?" Athletes in general have a difficult time staying down for any period. I felt so much comfort, and time was not the enemy by any means. It was an opportunity for me to enjoy some downtime. The two weeks went by fast, and I was able to spend my next two weeks in the media room, where I continued to pound away on this book. I was surprised at how much information was in my head that I could put to paper. I knew it was my time to write this book. I was excited to write a little each day.

All while writing this book, I had the best nurse. My husband took advantage of an offer to retire one year early after having served for thirty-two years, and we had had no idea the aforementioned surgery was coming. I was blessed with having him home full time and assisting me all the way in my recovery, which would not have been so easy without him providing everything I needed. I was mostly worried about good nutrition, and he took over with that right where I left off. I was amazed with his skills and desire to feed me to help me heal.

On December 21, we got to make the long drive back to Santa Monica to have my second post-surgery appointment. I was looking forward to seeing the doctor, but the drive frightened me. The thought of sitting in the car for hours on end was kind of a nightmare. We just pillowed up, and I was coming off the pain pills, but that day we added more. I had tried to lower my pain meds once about four days after the surgery, and that had turned into some unwanted pain rather swiftly, so I knew it wasn't time.

We always were so blessed driving to Santa Monica. We figured out a good time to drive down there without engaging in traffic. We made it in record time, only to discover Randy had left the crutches at home. He was beside himself, but I told him it would be OK and to just go in and borrow a pair of crutches. He left, and once he returned, he came with a wheelchair. I was upset because I wanted the doctor and nurses to see how well I was doing using crutches. Crutches are not easy to use, as they require a lot of upper-body strength. How do people without upper-body strength use them? But that wasn't a weakness of mine anymore.

I am always looking for some validation from the world, the kind that gets you into trouble. The doctor gave me a good report and told me to come back in six weeks. I would have my leg brace off by then, and physical therapy would be in full swing. It was a great feeling to get a good report, but it was also depressing to know that we were in no way out of the woods. A lot more time was going to need to come and pass. This meant that my positive attitude needed to stay, and I seriously needed to use common sense and self-control. I kept focusing on how blessed I was to have a good surgeon and how he had been willing to go the extra mile with me. I had told myself that this hamstring would be stronger than before. It had to have had some weakness in it, and that's why it had snapped. I was remembering that my powerlifting lift numbers never came back nearly as high as they had been when I started CrossFit. I had thought it was because of my age. Now I thought that it was because of a weakness and more than likely an injury already there. That thought gave me hope. Now that the injury was repaired, and if the repair held, perhaps it would be different with these lifts in the future. The thought of never being able to lift heavy again was something I had to keep suppressing, because lifting heavy was not coming anytime soon.

On January 1, we started to change the degrees on the leg brace to begin the straightening process of the leg and mainly the tendons. Little pains would come and go each time we would lessen the bend. Tweaks behind the knee, arch of my foot, inner thigh—they were all there telling me my leg was alive and well, just not used to working. It was a gradual descent, and I was ready to have that brace off and go on to physical therapy.

It was hard to have a good attitude coming into physical therapy this time because I had been assigned so much of it before—and all for nothing, maybe even worsening the situation by helping those ten-dons slide down farther as all that time passed. I had to go in with no anger and treat it as a new beginning. That's what I chose. The physi-cal therapy in the beginning, as the doctor had stated, would be very minimal, and indeed it was. After I met with the therapist a few times, she determined that I would be able to do most of it on my own for the first six weeks. I would be meeting with her only a few times, as there was not much to it. This worked out great. She also allowed me to walk a lot. I started out walking small bits and worked up to walking hills for up to an hour. Then, I would do physical therapy, which lasted about forty to fifty minutes, and then move on to upper-body movement. It felt so good to have some freedom again and begin to move and get my body back on the right track. I was getting plenty of exercise—nearly two hours per day.

Not long after I finished my physical therapy, which lasted three months, the surgeon released me, and I was on my own again for fitness. I started programming for myself with lifts, gymnastics skills, and met-cons. The doctor had reminded me that the improvements in running would be slow, and he didn't want me running for six to eight months, but that was fine because I could only jog anyway. My left leg would not allow me to run. With all the atrophy and reconstruction, it was akin to running with a stump, but it was changing for the better each day.

I had to start all my lifts very light, and I took advantage of that and worked on technique. I also hired a private instructor to work with me a few hours each week with Pilates. This was a smart move. She had her own studio, which included specialized equipment that would remove or add body weight. Removing the resistance in the beginning for me was great, considering the fact that I was recovering from a surgery. These apparatuses also helped put me into positions where I could increase my ROM in a way that I could not do it alone. I think this training was a big piece of my successful recovery. The breathing added another dimension for building the core and pelvic floor. For me, the most valuable parts of this training were achieving a higher level of ROM and the effects of oxygenating myself through breathing techniques.

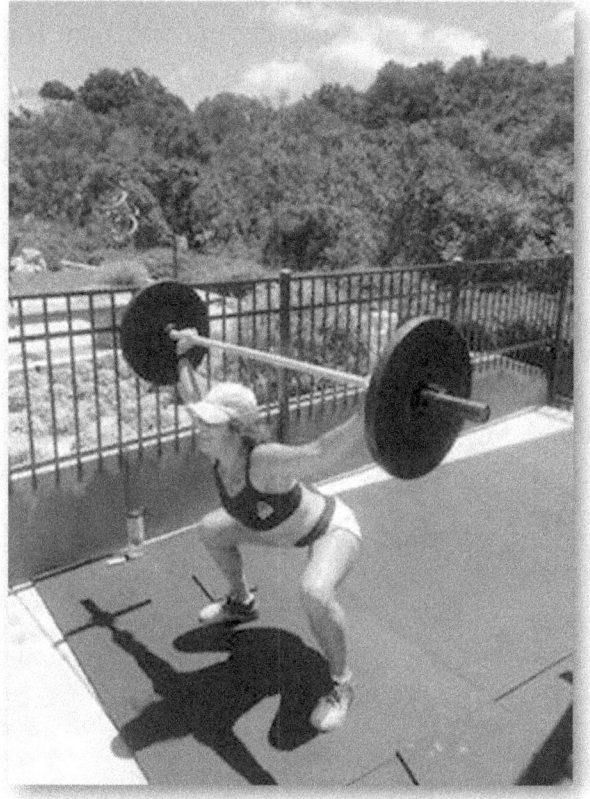

Rehabilitating the hamstring.

It has been ten months since that surgery day, and all my lifts are up to least 75 percent in all categories, if not more. I took my time and added five to ten pounds each week. This required discipline to hold back to the timetable, even when certain body parts and lifts were capable of putting more weight on sooner. The jogging has now become mediocre running. I still have a lot more work to do, but mainly time is the key. I have more advanced moves to master again, such as pistols and handstand walks, but I am satisfied with how things are working in that leg now. It will all come together eventually.

My recovery is successful because I listened to my doctor and did what he told me to do. I worked hard with my physical therapist and did what she said. I was patient and still am, but things could have gone differently if I had been on a true decondition plan from the get-go after the games. A rest period of several days would have been in that plan, as well as some light activity, followed by some light lifting and easy metcons. An example of that would be completing several identical before-games workouts with light work several days per week. Some light metcons, active rest, and mobility are what I would prescribe to anyone finishing heavy training and competition rather than cold-turkey rest. I believe that helps the mind, the hormones, and the physical body as well. This prevents injury.

Having an injury is a great way to spread the horizon of learning by taking something negative and turning it into something positive. Adding an injury chapter to this book has been golden, and what the injury taught me is priceless.

CHAPTER 19

EXERCISE FOR LIFE

WE KNOW THERE are many ways to move and stay fit. No matter which format you choose to move in, consistency is the key to staying fit, along with a healthy nutrition plan and daily detoxifying. Finding the appropriately challenging exercise plan that fits your schedule, mind, and body will provide longevity. I have been in the fitness world for over thirty years and have watched fitness and nutrition evolve. For the longest time, the emphasis was on long, bone-jarring cardio sessions, and the nutrition part was complex carbs. CrossFit has shone the light on intensity training. Their dedicated focus to strength training and gymnastics has enticed other fitness programs to add CrossFit into their regimens. Some of their rewards include well-rounded athletes, winning teams, and fewer injuries. Unlike many exercise programs in the past, CrossFit has implemented a solid nutrition program that should be everyone's lifestyle choice of eating in today's day and age. I think CrossFit is here to stay, along with many other wonderful exercise plans. I love that you can also compete in this sport! Implementing CrossFit into the school districts would be amazing!

Here are some things to consider if you decide to compete in your fitness arena. Compete for yourself, against yourself, and for your own improvements. This is far more satisfying, and the only pressure you have is the pressure you put on yourself. It's your choice whether you choose to compete. After competing in the games in 2015, I felt immensely satisfied with my results. Making the podium was my dream after 2013, and it finally happened. Of course, I had thoughts of winning it, but really my dream and therefore goal was to make the podium. When that came true, it felt like the end of my CrossFit-competing career for me. People asked me a question over and over: "Will you go back and compete at the games again?" I do not have regrets as to how much time I spent training and giving up family time. I would not go back and trade the experience at this point, but it sure felt as if it was time to move on after taking the bronze medal for the United States.

Indeed it was. I realized the other things in my life that I wanted to spend my time with. I also thought about how fortunate I was to be in those positions to compete at the games twice and how I could help others reach their fitness goals and manage health challenges, nutrition plans, and personal growth by focusing on them rather than my own competitions. If you think about it, we're all in some sort of a position where we can help others out, and I challenge you to put that in the forefront of your mind as you finish this book. I am still piecing together and finding the areas where I can help others. I know it's exactly what God wants from me, but I also continue to learn new things from others. Life never stops teaching. Seize each and every day!

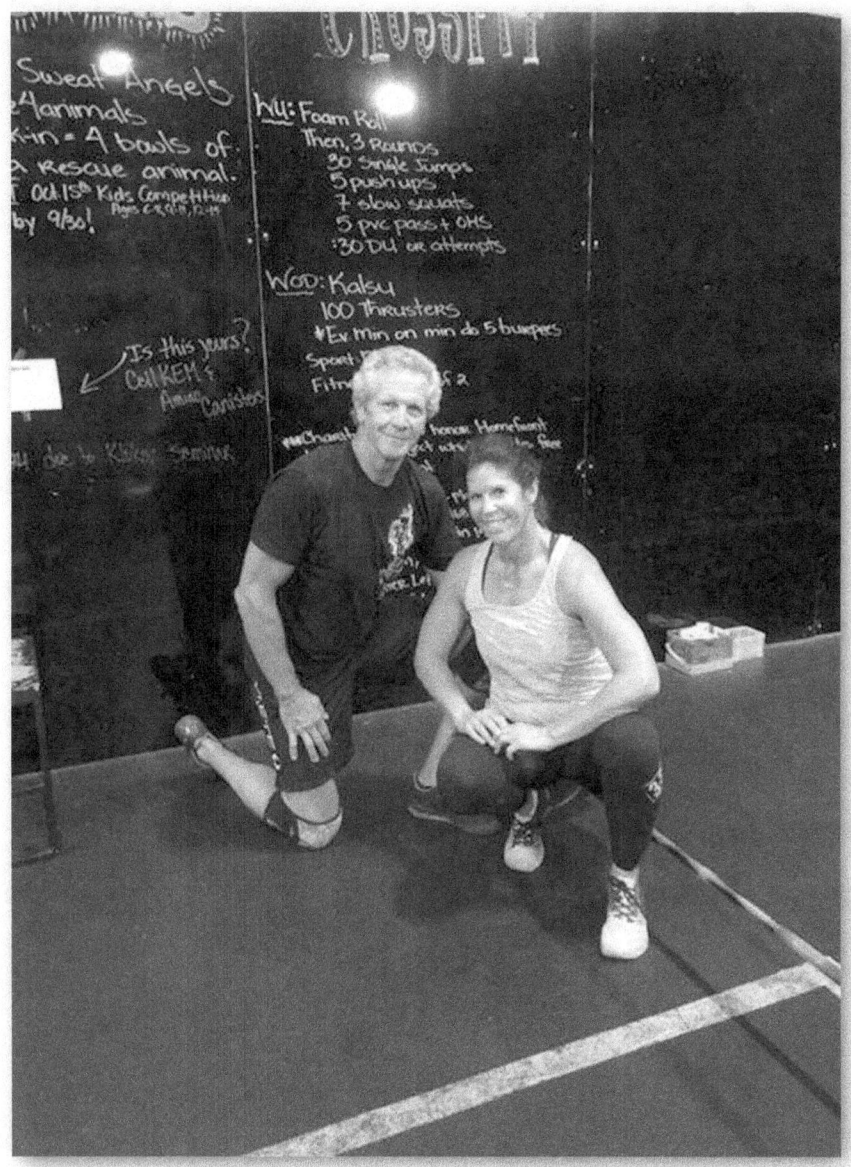

Completed hero WOD Kalsu at Iron Bar Crossfit
in Washington for PTSD benefit.

GLOSSARY

AMRAP: As Many Rounds As Possible in a given time allotment

Box: A gym or studio for CrossFit

C2B: Chest-to-bar pull-ups

Functional Medicine: Helps doctors and nurses implement personalized medicine; proactive and predictive; urges patients to become active in the their own health

GMO: Genetically modified organism

Kipping: A form of the word *kip*, which is a transference of movement first generated in the horizontal plane to the vertical plane, where momentum and a perfectly timed pull from the back launch the athlete forcefully upward

Metcon: Metabolic conditioning, a staple of CrossFit-style training

MUP: Muscle-up, a gymnastics movement done on rings

OLY: Olympic lifting

PR: Personal record

ROM: Range of motion

RX: Prescribed training program without scaling of weight or movement

Snatch: Olympic overhead lift

Thrusters: A two-part weight lifting movement with the weight lifting bar being pushed overhead from a squat

Triplet: Three movements in a WOD

WOD: Workout of the day

ABOUT THE AUTHOR

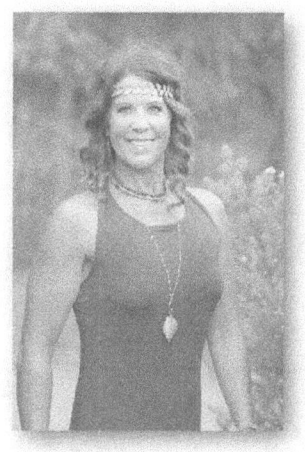

MICHELLE IS A devout Christian who lives in Arroyo Grande, a beautiful area of the central coast of California, with her husband, Randy, and her quarter horse, Roze of Sharon. Michelle has one daughter, Gabrieal, who is a paralegal in Redding, California, and three stepchildren residing in Alaska and Oklahoma. Michelle graduated from the University of Alaska at Anchorage with a bachelor's of science in physical education. She obtained five CrossFit certifications as she embarked on her CrossFit Master's career. She accomplished a thirteenth-place world finish in 2013 and a podium finish of the bronze medal in 2015 at the CrossFit Games in Los Angeles, California. She has been an entrepreneur nearly all her life, with the tendency to help others. Her quest to educate and help others achieve their health goals is her primary concern.